To my husband Gordon,
thanks for being so supportive

Acknowledgements

I would like to thank Claire Plimmer for commissioning this title. I'd also like to thank Simone Ryder, Founder of SWIB (Supporting Women in Business), for kindly agreeing to write the foreword. I'm also grateful to Anna Martin and Elanor Clarke for their very helpful editorial input.

Other titles in the Personal Health Guides series include:

50 Things You Can Do Today To Manage Anxiety
50 Things You Can Do Today To Manage Arthritis
50 Things You Can Do Today To Manage Back Pain
50 Things You Can Do Today To Manage Eczema
50 Things You Can Do Today To Manage Fibromyalgia
50 Things You Can Do Today To Increase Fertility
50 Things You Can Do Today To Manage Hay Fever
50 Things You Can Do Today To Manage IBS
50 Things You Can Do Today To Manage Insomnia
50 Things You Can Do Today To Manage Menopause
50 Things You Can Do Today To Manage Migraines
50 Things You Can Do Today To Boost Your Self-Esteem
50 Things You Can Do Today To Manage Stress

Contents

1. Learn about confidence

2. Eat fewer refined foods
3. Avoid too much alcohol
4. Cut down on caffeine
5. Eat more wholesome foods
6. Learn about key vitamins and minerals for good health
7. Get the exercise habit

8. Simplify your life
9. Take control of your spending
10. Cut work-related pressures
11. Change your attitude towards a stressful situation
12. Focus on the present

Author's Note

Fifteen years ago I decided to expand my horizons by studying for a BSc honours degree in health studies. I had been interested in health since my teens and felt it would be a very interesting topic to learn about and eventually write about. Aiming to gain a degree felt way outside my comfort zone and I was apprehensive. What if I found the course too difficult and failed to pass the modules and was asked to leave? What if I couldn't fit studying around caring for my teenage son and daughter? Despite my fears I went ahead and enrolled on the course. Throughout my studies I had niggling worries about failing or not being able to cope, but I kept going, encouraged by the marks I was achieving in my coursework and exams. With each success my confidence grew and at the end of three years of hard work I gained a first-class degree.

With my newfound confidence I decided to enrol on a Teaching in Further Education course to expand my employment opportunities. Again, I felt nervous – I found the idea of standing up and teaching daunting – but I told myself that if I could pass a degree course I could also gain a teaching certificate.

When I delivered my first micro-teach to fellow students I was so nervous I could barely speak, and when I did my first teaching practice delivering a seminar at a local university I froze when I stood up and addressed the students in the lecture theatre. However, each time I stretched my comfort zone I became a little more confident, until eventually I thought nothing of standing up and delivering lessons to adult learners of all ages and abilities.

What I have found is that when you aim higher you do feel a little uncomfortable initially, but if you go ahead despite your fears, your confidence will grow and your comfort zone will gradually become bigger and bigger. If you combine this philosophy with looking after your health and appearance, so that you feel and look your best, your confidence really can soar.

Wendy Green

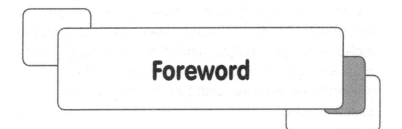

Foreword

by Simone Ryder, Founder of SWIB (Supporting Women in Business), Professional Coach, Author and Trainer in Confidence and Self-Empowerment

What a great book! Wendy has touched a subject very close to my heart. Having struggled to be confident enough to be myself and express who I am in the past, I now meet and support many women in my work, helping them feel empowered and confident in both work and life.

Many years ago as a single mum, very overweight and unhealthy, I had little confidence in myself. However, as Wendy suggests in her book, being body-confident can really increase your self-esteem; so I set goals and began to look after my health, and as I lost weight my confidence increased too. I like the way this book focuses on wellbeing, because this is where my success first started, and when my confidence increased I found ways to make all my dreams come true.

How to do this is the question and I can relate to this well. I know from my own experience of going back into education as a mature student with two daughters to bring up, starting a business on my own, writing a book and losing a lot of weight, that whatever the goal, the key has always been a deep-down feeling that I won't give up on what is important to me; this is the place where your inner confidence is developed, and Wendy encourages you and shows you how to develop this discipline within yourself.

In the chapter about building your confidence through complementary therapies you will find suggestions of how to support yourself, nurturing your mind, body and soul to stay calm and focused, and therefore more able to cope confidently.

Trying things for the first time is scary; for me going into business meetings, presenting and networking with strangers made me a bag of nerves when I first started out, but I needed to look confident and I soon found that wearing the right, smart clothes, being well groomed and well prepared, as Wendy suggests, helped me a lot. It was a bit like acting, but these techniques see you through until you really do feel strong inside.

Ultimately, I have found that confidence comes from being true to yourself and finding the right mix of strategies to help you grow in strength as a person, staying calm and grounded in your mind and heart about who you are and how you express yourself. Wendy has provided this wonderful toolbox of techniques, strategies and suggestions in her book to help you achieve the confidence you need to feel how you want to feel and succeed in life.

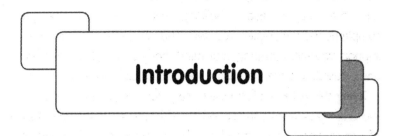

Introduction

Strong self-confidence enables you to be successful and achieve your full potential in every area of your life, whereas a lack of confidence can hold you back. This book explains what confidence is, as well as what affects it, and offers practical advice and a holistic approach to help you boost yours.

Good physical and mental health are the cornerstones of confidence – it's hard to feel good about yourself if you feel unfit or unwell, or if you are suffering from low mood; Chapter 2 offers you tips on eating well and becoming more active, while Chapter 3 covers stress management and how to sleep more soundly.

Negative thoughts can cripple your self-confidence, so in Chapter 4 we look at how you can change the way you think about yourself to create unshakeable self-belief. Many people who appear confident confess to acting as if they're confident even when they don't feel it; Chapter 5 explains how you can feel more confident simply by adopting the body language, voice and vocabulary of a confident person.

Doing the things you're good at is a great confidence-booster, so Chapter 6 encourages you to identify and develop your innate talents. Your confidence grows when you take action, so Chapter 7 encourages you to step out of your comfort zone and do the things you fear to help you develop strong self-belief. Chapter 8 looks at how you can boost your confidence by acknowledging your past successes and building on them by setting and achieving new goals; there are also sections on how to use affirmations and visualisations to boost your confidence and your chances of success in any situation.

Knowing that you are looking your best is also an important aspect of feeling confident, so in Chapter 9 you will find effective grooming and style tips. Feeling relaxed and pampered can do wonders for your general wellbeing and therefore help you feel more confident; Chapter 10 offers a selection of relaxing techniques and treatments from complementary therapies you can try for yourself. Chapter 11 suggests how you can apply the techniques and ideas from this book to real-life situations that often challenge even the most confident person. At the end of the book you'll find recipes based on the dietary guidelines, as well as details of helpful products, books and organisations.

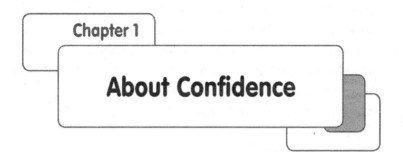

Chapter 1

About Confidence

In this chapter we will consider what confidence is and how it differs from self-esteem, as well as the factors that can affect your confidence.

1. Learn about confidence

What is confidence?

In simple terms, confidence is having a strong belief in yourself and your ability to achieve your goals. Being positive about yourself and optimistic about the future are also important aspects of feeling confident. Confidence empowers you to go for what you want in life, while a lack of it can leave you stuck in a rut and frightened of making positive changes.

However, confidence is not about having an over-inflated view of yourself, or about being arrogant and putting other people down to make yourself feel better. When you are truly confident you should feel so comfortable in your own skin that you don't need to show off, or belittle other people to make yourself look good.

What is the difference between self-esteem and confidence?

Self-esteem and confidence are often used interchangeably, but there are differences between the two concepts; self-esteem is how you rate or appraise yourself as a person, whereas confidence is about how much faith you have in your abilities and how you project yourself to others.

What affects confidence?

Your confidence can be affected by a number of things, including your personality, i.e. whether you are an extrovert or introvert, your mental and physical health, and the beliefs you have developed about yourself throughout your life in response to your experiences and relationships at home, at school, at work and in your personal life.

Examples of events and experiences that may have affected your self-confidence include:

Your upbringing – did your parents encourage you and praise you when you did something well?

Your experiences at school – were you bullied by your peers or given negative feedback by a teacher?

Divorce/end of a relationship – when a relationship ends your confidence can take a knock – especially if your partner has left you.

Bereavement – coping with the loss of a loved one can leave you feeling physically and mentally drained, which in turn chips away at your confidence.

Physical ill-health – having to deal with illness can sap your energy and your belief in your ability to cope with life's challenges.

 Depression/anxiety – low mood and anxiety are linked to negative thinking, which can have a disastrous effect on your self-confidence.

 Dissatisfaction with the way you look – feeling unhappy about your appearance – for example, if you are overweight or suffer from bad skin – can leave you lacking confidence in all areas of your life.

 Redundancy/unemployment – losing your job can deliver a huge blow to your confidence in your abilities.

 Workplace bullying – being the victim of workplace bullying can take its toll on your performance at work, which can in turn make you feel less confident in your ability to do your job.

 Relocating – this means you have to start afresh – possibly starting a new job and having to make new friends, both of which can challenge even the most confident of people.

 Having a baby – being at home full-time with a baby and all that it can entail, e.g. sleepless nights and social isolation, can dent your self-confidence; juggling a full-time job with parenthood can leave you exhausted, which can also sap your confidence.

 Excessive pressure (stress) – if you feel overwhelmed by too much pressure, your performance and mental and physical health are likely to be negatively affected, all of which can lower your self-confidence.

How can I become more confident?

The good news is that no matter whether you are an introvert or an extrovert, or how past experiences and relationships have affected you, it is possible to boost your self-confidence.

You can cultivate strong self-confidence by taking good care of your physical and mental health; challenging negative thoughts and beliefs about yourself; identifying and developing your natural talents by setting and achieving realistic goals, and stepping out of your comfort zone. Ensuring you look the part by holding yourself well, watching your body language and making the most of your appearance can also help build your self-confidence. Improving your general wellbeing with techniques from complementary therapies such as the Alexander Technique, aromatherapy and the emotional freedom techniques (EFT) could also have a positive effect on your self-belief. This book offers you practical advice in each of these areas to help you develop genuine, long-lasting self-confidence.

Are you an extrovert or an introvert?

We all have an extroverted and introverted side, but one is usually more dominant than the other.

Extroverts are sociable, talkative, assertive and outgoing, and tend to think out loud and on their feet.

Introverts typically prefer less-stimulating environments, tend to focus on their private thoughts and feelings, listen more than they talk and think before they speak.

Although an extrovert might appear to have a head start in the confidence stakes, it is still possible to be a confident introvert; this book can help you to change how you think and feel and become more assertive to boost your confidence.

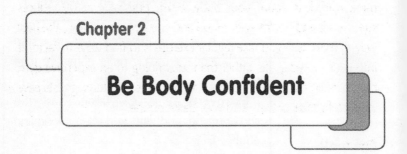

Chapter 2

Be Body Confident

Good physical and psychological health are vital if you want to feel confident. Eating well, taking regular exercise, managing stress and taking steps to ensure you get sufficient good quality sleep will mean that you look and feel great and have boundless energy. Looking and feeling your best will give you strong foundations on which to build unshakeable self-confidence. All of these aspects of health are inter-related; a poor diet and lack of exercise can lead to stress and poor sleep – both of which could affect your confidence negatively. Suffering from stress and poor sleep can make you more likely to crave fatty, sugary, salty, processed foods and less inclined to take regular exercise, which could lead to weight gain and poor health – which again are likely to have a negative impact on self-confidence. We look at the effects of stress and lack of sleep on confidence in more detail in Chapter 3.

Eating well shouldn't be about depriving yourself of your favourite foods, but more about enjoying tasty meals made from wholesome, nutritious ingredients, rather than over-refined and processed foods. At the beginning of this chapter you will find easy-to-follow advice on tweaking your diet to make sure you get all the nutrients you need for a healthy mind and body, while still enjoying what you eat. At the end of the book you will find some delicious wholesome recipes that incorporate these healthy eating guidelines.

As well as improving your physical health and helping you to feel more confident about your body, being physically active reduces stress levels and boosts both mood and energy levels. Often, the best way to make sure you take regular exercise is to find ways to factor it into your everyday life, rather than subscribing to an expensive gym membership that you are unlikely to use; this chapter suggests easy ways to fit more activity into your daily routine.

Eat well

There are a lot of fad diets around, all promising to give you the perfect body; low-fat, low-carbohydrate, high-protein... the list is endless. However, to ensure you get all the nutrients you need for good health, the best advice is to avoid cutting out any particular food group; low-fat diets have been linked to depression and skin conditions like eczema; low-carbohydrate and high-protein diets have been associated with low energy, constipation, high cholesterol and even kidney damage. Also, such diets are usually impossible to stick to long term and most people regain any weight they have lost when they revert back to their normal eating habits. Not only that, but when you severely restrict your calorie intake your body adapts by slowing down your metabolism, so when you eventually increase your food intake you gain even more weight and find it harder to lose weight in the future.

Instead, aim to eat a healthy, balanced diet that includes all the different food groups to help you manage your weight and enjoy good physical and mental health. This will boost your confidence in general, as well as help you to feel better about your body and appearance.

Processed foods like cakes, biscuits, sweets, white bread, pies, pizzas, crisps and ready meals are generally low in disease-preventing fibre, vitamins and minerals, and contain hidden nasties like sugar, salt, saturated fats, trans fats, artificial sweeteners, colourings and preservatives, which in excess are linked to weight gain, type 2 diabetes, high blood pressure, heart disease and stroke.

The key to good nutrition is to go back to basics, which means cutting back on refined, sugary, salty, processed foods and alcohol, and eating more wholesome, unrefined foods.

Aim to eat only when you are hungry and stop when you're full. It is best not to 'ban' any particular food as it is human nature to want what you think you can't have; instead try to eat everything in moderation and to develop a taste for healthier foods, so that you can still satisfy your palate while managing your weight.

If you comfort eat to cope with stress and negative emotions such as anger or hurt, look for ways to express and deal with your feelings, such as talking them through with someone you trust, or writing them down. Identify any underlying issues or problems and seek solutions, so that you start treating food as fuel for your body, rather than a means of escaping from your emotions. Try to eat slowly and focus on the sight, smell, taste and texture of your food. What you are doing is gradually building a healthy relationship with food that will enable you to achieve a healthy weight in the long term.

Portion caution

Reducing your portion sizes is an important part of eating healthily; even if you eat wholesome foods, if you consume too much of them you will gain weight. Try eating from a smaller plate to automatically cut your portion size and trick your brain into thinking you've eaten a lot.

2. Eat fewer refined foods

Refined, processed foods are likely to be low in fibre, vitamins and minerals, and high in sugar, salt, and saturated and trans fats.

 Refined carbohydrates – such as white bread, pastries, sugary drinks and sweets, are digested quickly, causing your blood sugar to rapidly rise and then fall. Low blood sugar leads to mood swings, poor concentration, fatigue and irritability, while excess sugar is linked to obesity and Type 2 diabetes. Choose wholegrain foods instead (see Action 5) and foods low in sugar; you can do this by checking the labels (see below). When cooking and baking you can often cut the amount of sugar by half without spoiling the quality of the finished product.

Salt – the current recommendation is that adults should eat no more than 6 g daily. Processed foods such as canned soups, frozen pizzas and ready meals often contain added salt; keep the intake of these to a minimum and where possible choose foods low in sodium (salt) by checking the label (see below). Use herbs and spices such as basil, rosemary, mint, garlic and chillies instead of salt when cooking and benefit from the disease-preventing antioxidants they contain, too.

Saturated fats – otherwise known as hard fats, are mainly found in animal products such as red meat, butter and full-fat dairy foods like cheese and milk, and in processed foods like pies, cakes, biscuits and ready meals A diet high in saturated fat is thought to raise 'bad' LDL cholesterol levels, which increases the risk of heart disease and atherosclerosis (hardening of the arteries); eat these foods sparingly and go for reduced-fat versions whenever possible, making sure you read the labels (see page 24).

◻ **Trans fats** – also known as partially hydrogenated fats, are solid fats manufactured from liquid vegetable oils using a process called hydrogenation. Trans fats tend to be used in some margarines and in processed foods like biscuits, pies and cakes to help extend their shelf life. Eating a lot of foods containing trans fats also raises LDL cholesterol levels.

Quick and easy guide to food labels

Ingredients, including additives, have to be listed in descending order of weight, so it's easy to spot the main ones. Some food manufacturers use traffic light colours on the front of their products to help identify if the food has low, medium or high levels of fat, sugar and salt. Green indicates low, amber medium and red high. So the more green lights something has the healthier it is, in terms of fat, sugar and salt levels.

Most food companies will provide nutritional information including the calories and grams of sugars, fats and salt in a serving of food, and how this measures up as a percentage of your guideline daily amounts (GDA). These are based on the energy and nutrient requirements of an average adult. One downside is that the figures given are often for smaller servings than most people eat. Also, people's dietary needs vary depending on their age, gender and activity level. However, the information can help you to make sensible food choices. As a general guide, 5 per cent or less of your GDA is low, whilst 20 per cent or more is high.

3. Avoid too much alcohol

Avoid the temptation to drink too much to hide a lack of confidence. Drinking excessive amounts of alcohol depletes B vitamins, calcium and magnesium – the very nutrients needed for a positive, confident outlook on life. Drinking alcohol to steady your nerves before a big event is definitely something to avoid; you could lose your inhibitions and end up saying or doing something you might regret later. Alcohol is also addictive and drinking to excess is linked to liver and heart disease, a number of cancers and diabetes, so stick to the recommended maximum weekly alcohol intake of 14 units for a woman and 21 units for a man. One unit roughly equates to one small (125 ml) glass of wine, half a pint of lager or bitter, one small glass of sherry or port, or one single measure of spirits. You should also aim to have at least two alcohol-free days a week. To find out more visit www.drinkaware.co.uk.

Enjoy a glass of red wine

A growing body of research suggests that drinking a glass of red wine a few times per week benefits health. The combination of alcohol and plant chemicals called procyanidins is thought to protect against atherosclerosis (furring up of the arteries) and blood clots, which are both major causes of heart disease and stroke. Cabernet Sauvignon, Chianti, Merlot and Pinot Noir are thought to be the most beneficial.

4. Cut down on caffeine

When consumed in moderation, caffeine boosts concentration and alertness, and may cut the risk of dementia. Drinks and foods that contain caffeine, i.e. coffee, tea, cola and chocolate, also provide beneficial antioxidants; however, heavy caffeine consumption has been linked to irritability, nervousness, restlessness and insomnia, none of which are conducive to feeling confident. So if you consume a lot of caffeine-containing drinks and foods, it may be worth cutting down.

The amount of caffeine in a cup of tea or coffee can vary quite a lot depending on the brand, how much tea or coffee is used, how long it's left to brew and, of course, the size of the cup or portion. Some people are more sensitive to caffeine than others, but experts suggest a daily limit of 300 mg; as a rough guide a cup of tea contains around 50 mg, whereas a cup of ground coffee contains around 100 mg; 50 g of dark chocolate contains up to 50 mg and the same amount of milk chocolate contains around 25 mg. Good alternatives to regular tea and coffee include decaffeinated versions, redbush (rooibos) tea, herbal teas and coffee substitutes made from dandelion (e.g. Symington's Dandelion Coffee) or chicory (e.g. Prewett's Instant Chicory). Always wean yourself off caffeine gradually to prevent withdrawal symptoms, which can include headaches and anxiety.

5. Eat more wholesome foods

Wholegrain carbohydrates – such as wholemeal or granary bread, brown rice, wholewheat pasta, porridge oats and barley. The bran which encases wholegrains means they take longer to digest, so the glucose they provide is released slowly for sustained energy, which aids weight management and helps prevent mood swings. They also provide B vitamins for a healthy nervous system.

Beans, peas and lentils – are good sources of protein, slow-release carbohydrate, soluble and insoluble fibre, vitamins and minerals. A serving counts as one portion of vegetables.

Fruit and vegetables – supply various vitamins, minerals, phytochemicals (plant chemicals) including antioxidants, and fibre, all of which benefit health in many ways, such as helping to prevent heart disease and certain cancers. Eat at least five portions a day in a rainbow of colours to get a wide range of nutrients. Satisfy sugar cravings with dried fruit such as raisins, sultanas, dates, figs, prunes and dried apricots, and fresh fruit such as bananas, melons and strawberries.

Nuts and seeds – provide essential fatty acids omega-3, 6 and 9 for brain and heart health, and healthy skin, hair and nails, as well as protein, minerals such as calcium and magnesium, fibre and vitamin E.

Lean proteins – such as chicken, turkey, fish, beef and pork with all visible fat trimmed off before cooking, or tofu and seitan (a meat substitute made from wheat protein) for vegetarians and vegans. These provide vital amino acids, the building blocks of life, including tryptophan and phenylalanine, which the brain uses to make the confidence-enhancing 'happy hormone' serotonin and 'motivating hormones' dopamine, noradrenaline and adrenaline. These are all known as neurotransmitters; brain chemicals which help to transmit messages throughout the nervous system. Proteins also help you to feel fuller for longer because they slow down the rate at which carbohydrates are absorbed, helping to balance mood and maintain a healthy weight. Eating protein-rich foods with wholegrains helps the brain to absorb the tryptophan and phenylalanine they contain.

Liver – is rich in vitamins A, B, C, and the minerals iron and selenium, making it a very nutritious food; it is best eaten just once or twice a week, due to its high cholesterol content.

Fish – especially oily fish like sardines, salmon and mackerel, as well as providing protein, supply omega-3 fats, which are essential for brain and heart health. They are also the best dietary source of vitamin D – a lack of which has been linked to various conditions including depression, joint and muscle pain, osteoporosis, poor immunity and certain cancers. Aim to eat oily fish twice a week.

Eggs – are another great source of protein and vitamins A, B, D and E, as well as the antioxidants lutein and zeaxanthin, which are thought to protect against two causes of sight loss in old age: cataracts and age-related macular degeneration (AMD).

Reduced-fat dairy products (including milk, yoghurt and cheese, or calcium-enriched soya alternatives) – are a good source of calcium for strong bones and teeth and a calm disposition. Yoghurt and mature cheeses such as Cheddar, Gouda, Emmental and blue cheeses contain probiotics ('good' bacteria) that keep the gut healthy and boost the immune system.

Olive and rapeseed oil – these lower low-density lipoprotein LDL (bad) cholesterol and raise high-density lipoprotein HDL (good) cholesterol. Use them in cooking and buy margarines that contain them to ensure you get the right balance of omega-3 and omega-6 fats in your diet.

Note: Remember all fats are high in calories, so to ensure a balanced diet and to help maintain a healthy weight it's recommended that no more than a third of our daily energy intake comes from fats. This equates to about 75 g for women, of which no more than 20 g should be saturated fat, and 90 g for men, of which no more than 30 g should be saturated fats.

Cocoa and dark (70 per cent cocoa and above) chocolate – are rich in antioxidants such as flavonols and procyanidins which are thought to prevent heart disease and stroke by widening the arteries, boosting HDL (good) cholesterol and lowering LDL (bad) cholesterol. They contain theobromine too, which has a gentle, stimulant effect on the brain. They also boost levels of the 'happy hormone' serotonin, so go on, treat yourself! However, dark chocolate also contains sugar and fat, so try to limit your intake to about 50 g a day.

Water – staying well hydrated is vital for mental and physical wellbeing, and helps to prevent overeating. Experts recommend 1.2–2.2 litres of water daily; this sounds like a lot, but remember fruit and vegetables contain a lot of water and can contribute to your daily intake. Tea and coffee count (they still contribute fluid, despite having a slight diuretic effect), but avoid drinking more than a few cups a day as they contain caffeine, too much of which can cause jitteriness and insomnia; see Action 4, Cut down on caffeine.

6. Learn about key vitamins and minerals for good health

Below is an overview of the key vitamins and minerals you need for good health.

Vitamin/mineral	Needed for	Good sources
Vitamin A (retinol from animal products and beta-carotene from fruit and vegetables)	Strong immunity; formation of new bone; healthy skin, hair and eyes.	Liver, cod or halibut-liver oils, eggs, dairy foods, spinach, carrots, apricots.
B vitamins	Good mental health; conversion of food into energy; healthy skin, eyes, nerves, muscles and heart. Shortage associated with depression.	Wholegrains, poultry, fish and nuts, meat, offal, most fruits and vegetables (especially dark-green leafy), eggs, dairy products and yeast extract.
Vitamin C	Immunity; wound healing; growth and maintenance of bones, teeth, gums, ligaments and blood vessels.	Blackcurrants, citrus fruits, berries, peppers (especially red), tomatoes, broccoli, kale, tomatoes, potatoes, peas and cabbage.

Vitamin D	Strong bones and teeth; good mental health; strong immunity. Lack of vitamin D linked to low mood and infections.	Best source is sun exposure. Food sources include fish-liver oils, oily fish, i.e. herring, pilchards, mackerel salmon and sardines, eggs, liver, butter, fortified margarines, cereals, milks and mushrooms.
Vitamin E	Protection against free radicals, normal growth and development; healthy immune system and blood vessels.	Berries (in the seeds), avocados, sweet potatoes, nuts, seeds, olive oil and wholegrains.
Vitamin K	Strong bones and blood clotting. A lack of vitamin K has been linked with osteoporosis and atherosclerosis (hardening of the arteries).	Broccoli, spinach, kale, sprouts, oats wholewheat cereals and olive oil.

Calcium	Strong bones and teeth; healthy nervous system; blood clotting and muscle contraction. Insufficient amounts can cause tenseness, irritability, difficulty relaxing and sleeping.	Low-fat milk, cheeses, especially Edam and hard cheeses like Parmesan and Padano, and yoghurt; calcium-fortified soya alternatives; tinned sardines (if you eat the bones), almonds, seeds, dried apricots, oranges, oats, Brazil nuts, molasses, watercress, leeks, parsnips, lentils, beans (especially red kidney beans), green leafy vegetables, broccoli, celery and tap water.
Chromium	Keeping blood sugar steady by working with insulin to remove excess glucose from the blood. Also involved in breakdown of fats.	Chicken, beef, liver, eggs, wholegrains, apples, bananas, tomatoes, green peppers, spinach, onions, lentils, herbs and spices.

Iron	Production of haemoglobin, which carries oxygen around the body. Lack of iron can lead to fatigue and low mood.	Liver, shellfish, sardines, meat, poultry, nuts, dried fruit (especially apricots), dark green leafy vegetables, beans, peas and lentils, wholegrain bread and cereals, muesli. Tip: drink a glass of orange juice when you eat these foods; the vitamin C helps iron absorption.
Magnesium	Bone growth; healthy nervous system and muscle function. Shortage can lead to depression.	Wholemeal bread, brown rice, bran or wholewheat cereals, oats, nuts and seeds, dark-green leafy vegetables, baked beans, peas, potatoes, fish, dairy foods and dark chocolate.

Selenium	Healthy nervous system; protects against free radical damage. Shortage is linked to low mood.	Wholegrains, eggs, fish, shellfish, meat, poultry, Brazil nuts, cashew nuts, sunflower seeds, lentils, wheat germ, garlic, mushrooms and brewer's yeast.
Zinc	Healthy nervous system; healing of wounds; cell growth and repair. Shortage is linked to low mood and lack of motivation.	Meat, fish and shellfish, such as oysters, mussels and prawns; eggs, dairy foods, wholegrains, nuts, seeds, beans, mushrooms, broccoli, squash, spinach, kiwi and blackberries.

7. Get the exercise habit

When it comes to being active it doesn't really matter what you do so long as you get your body moving. The problem with modern-day living is that it is all too easy to be inactive. We have more labour-saving devices in the home than our parents and grandparents did, and it's easy to jump in the car even for short journeys when you could walk. An ever-growing number of us have sedentary jobs that involve sitting at a desk for long periods of time; and as a nation two of our favourite pastimes – watching TV and using the Internet – involve sitting down for hours on end.

The current recommendations are that we take moderate exercise, such as brisk walking or mowing the lawn, for at least half an hour five times a week; but try to think of this as the bare minimum; exercising more than this will help ensure that you are at the peak of physical fitness and help prevent life-threatening conditions like type 2 diabetes, heart disease, stroke, dementia and breast, bowel and other cancers, as well as boost mood and build stronger bones and muscles. If by now you are thinking: but I haven't got time to exercise, think again. With a little thought and ingenuity it is possible to transform yourself from couch potato to fit and active.

Here are some ideas to get you started and I'm sure you'll think of more.

At work

◯ Park your car further from your workplace.

◯ Get off the bus or train one stop earlier.

◯ Park your car on the top level of a multi-storey car park and use the stairs down and back up.

◯ Use the stairs rather than the lift.

◯ Use a pedal pusher exerciser; place it under your desk and you can pedal away as you work.

◯ Take a walk during your lunch break, instead of sitting at your desk.

◯ Walk to your colleagues' desks to pass on information instead of emailing them.

◯ Walk to the water dispenser or tap every hour or two for a refill; your brain will benefit from both the exercise and the extra hydration.

◯ Make regular trips to the kitchen to make a tea or coffee.

At home

◯ Be a domestic goddess/god; vacuuming, dusting and cleaning not only gives the body a good workout but, according to research published in the *British Journal of Sports Medicine* in 2008, also reduces the risk of suffering from anxiety and depression.

◯ Walk your dog every day, or if you don't have one, offer to walk a neighbour's.

◯ Use a cordless or mobile phone so you can walk as you talk.

◯ Wash the car by hand; it's probably just as quick as driving round to the car wash and much better for your fitness levels.

◯ Park your car further away from the shops if you are only buying a few items.

◯ Use a basket, rather than a trolley, whenever you only need a few groceries.

◯ If your children's school is within walking distance, stop the school run and walk instead.

Take your baby or toddler to the park; pushing a pram or buggy is great exercise for you and is a great way to settle a fretful baby or a bored or over-tired toddler.

If you have older children, play ball games in the garden, take them for a long walk, or visit your local swimming pool.

Get gardening; even doing light gardening tasks can increase your strength and agility and improve muscle tone.

Try rebounding

If you can't get outdoors try using a rebounder. This is a mini-trampoline that is ideal for home use. Research suggests that rebounding not only boosts fitness and mood, but also improves posture, balance and co-ordination. Just put on some music and march for a minute or two to warm up, then bounce for a couple of minutes, before marching again for a further few minutes. For more information go to www.rebound-uk.com.

Chapter 3

Control Stress for Strong Self-Confidence

A little pressure can be challenging and stimulating, and help push us to achieve our full potential – without it we'd lack the motivation to get out of bed each morning; most of us would find a life without any kind of pressure boring, and boredom can be stressful in itself. Each of us have individual levels and types of pressure we feel comfortable with; what is challenging and motivating for one person might be completely overwhelming for another. Psychologists argue that stress arises from your perception of a situation, rather than from the situation itself, so changing the way you view events can help you to reduce stress.

Too much pressure in our lives leads to stress and, left unchecked, stress can cause chemical changes in the body that can eventually lead to health problems ranging from irritability, anxiety, weight gain, skin conditions, migraines, IBS, aches and pains, colds and flu, to depression, high blood pressure, irregular heartbeat and heart disease. Suffering from any of these physical and emotional problems could seriously undermine your self-confidence. Also, when you are under excessive pressure you are more likely to feel unsure of yourself and perform less well, which in turn depletes your confidence in your abilities.

As a nation we experience more stress than ever before because we are increasingly aspirational and materialistic, which makes our lives ever more complex; we have far more services and products to choose from; the media and advertisers constantly bombard us with images of slim, attractive people in designer clothes, driving top-of-the-range cars and living in big houses, full of material goods like widescreen TVs and the latest technology. This type of lifestyle is unattainable for most of us, yet the way it is presented to us leaves us feeling we must strive to achieve it either by working increasingly longer hours or running up debt.

If you lack confidence you might be tempted to buy things you don't need to compensate, which can lead to spiralling debts. Worrying about debt and how to make ends meet is exhausting and eats away at your self-confidence, leading to a vicious cycle of low self-confidence and debt. The best way to break the cycle is to work on boosting your self-confidence by following some of the tips in this book and taking control of your finances.

Many of us juggle full or part-time work with parenthood, a relationship and running a home, whilst trying to look and feel our best and maintain a social life. Stress is now the most common reason for British workers to be signed off on long-term sick leave and work itself can be a major cause of stress. A report by the Institute of Personnel & Development in 2011 cited job insecurity caused by the economic downturn, an excessive workload, poor management and restructuring in the workplace as the leading causes of work-related stress. Other factors include lack of control over your work situation, working long hours or shifts, not having time to take breaks, or having too much responsibility. Lack of help and support from your co-workers or supervisors, having no opportunities to advance, and doing a job that is boring and repetitive can also take their toll.

Stress is also a major cause of sleep problems, including difficulty falling asleep and staying asleep, and lack of sleep can trigger the stress response, creating a vicious cycle of stress and insomnia. Clearly stress can have a serious negative impact on your physical and mental health, therefore managing it should be considered an integral part of both raising and maintaining self-confidence.

In this chapter we look at how simplifying your life, taking control of your spending, cutting work-related pressures, changing your attitude towards challenging situations and taking time out to relax can cut the amount of stress you experience. In the final section you will find some tips to help you sleep soundly.

8. Simplify your life

The more you can simplify your life, the less stressed you will feel. Try living by these rules:

Prioritise – identify the three most important tasks you must do today and do them first. Say 'no' to non-essential tasks you don't have time for, or just don't want to do.

Delegate – if you share a house with others, make sure everyone does their fair share of the chores. Discuss who should do what and, if necessary, draw up a weekly rota and stick it on the fridge or in another prominent place.

De-clutter – to save time and energy, and feel calmer and more in control, if you haven't worn, read or used an item for two years or more put it into one of three piles: 'bin it', 'donate to charity' and 'recycle or sell it'; recycle goods through Freegle, Freecycle or Clothes for Cash (see Directory), or sell them on eBay; swap or sell unwanted clothes on www.bigwardrobe.com. Ditch toiletries and cosmetics past their use-by date.

Take the stress out of cleaning – only tackle a couple of rooms at a time. Clean the dirtiest room first. Clean first then vacuum. Wear an apron with pockets, so that you can keep your cleaning products, cloths and dusters handy. Clean from left to right, top to bottom and from the back of an item to the front – without doubling back. Only clean dirty areas, i.e. don't clean a whole door; just wipe away any visible marks.

Keep your home tidy

Once you've cleared the clutter, try these tips to stop it building up again:

1. Keep a waste bin in every room.

2. Bin or recycle newspapers and letters you don't need to keep as soon as you have read them.

3. Ensure you have plenty of cupboards, boxes, baskets and shelves for storage.

4. Ask everyone in the house to tidy up after themselves.

5. Use up existing toiletries, cosmetics, cleaning products, etc. before buying new ones.

6. De-clutter at least once a year.

Avoid information overload – be selective about your TV viewing; only watch what really interests you. Switch your mobile phone off in the evening and make the dining room and bedroom text-free areas. Only check personal emails twice a day; ensure the spam filter is on and as soon as you have answered an email, file it in a folder or delete it. Set yourself a daily time limit for online browsing and only answer the Twitter or Facebook messages you want to respond to. This will also increase the amount of deep restorative sleep you get because your brain won't have as much information to process during sleep.

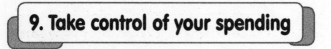

9. Take control of your spending

Avoid the stress of debt problems by taking control of your spending.

Work out how much money you need to cover your essential outgoings

Figure out how many outgoing payments you make a month, such as mortgage/rent, gas, electricity, food, insurance and travel, then set a realistic budget and stick to it. Check if you can save money by switching your mortgage lender or energy supplier, and pay your energy bills by direct debit for the cheapest deal.

Identify your money wasters

Keep a spending diary for a month to see where you are wasting your hard-earned cash, then vow to only buy the things you really want and need. Check your direct debits and standing orders to see if you're paying for something you don't need and could cancel – for example, insurance on goods you no longer have, a subscription to a magazine you never read, an unused gym membership, or an 'added value' bank account you pay extra for but don't use the additional benefits, such as mobile phone insurance, or credit card protection.

Pay off any debts as soon as possible

If you are struggling to meet credit card or mortgage payments, speak to your lender as soon possible to negotiate an amount you can manage to pay. Pay off the debts with the highest rates first. If you are in serious debt through credit and store cards you need to take drastic action – cut them up now!

Spend your money on your priorities

Rather than spending your money on things you don't really need or want simply to meet social expectations, or in an attempt to boost your confidence, think about what is most important to you and then spend your money accordingly. For example, if you enjoy going on holiday a couple of times a year, maybe you could direct more of your money towards your travel costs by cutting out another major expense, such as running a car; perhaps you could manage without if your local public transport services are adequate or if you could cycle or walk to work.

Live more frugally

Doing this will enable you to spend less, but still afford the things you enjoy.

- Before you buy anything ask: Do I need it? Will I use/wear it? Does it suit me? Can I buy it somewhere else for less?

- If you buy the more expensive brands, bear in mind that you are often paying for their higher advertising and packaging costs.

- If you spend a lot of money on eating out, limit it to a weekly treat and make the most of local 'early-bird' deals, eat at your local college restaurant and check daily deals sites for money-saving vouchers to use at local eateries.

◯ Use your local library or swap books with friends when you have read them. Alternatively, register with a book-swapping website such as www.readitswapit.co.uk, or use www.bookcrossing.com

◯ Check online for the cheapest holiday deals; all-inclusive deals tend to be the most cost effective as you don't have to worry about how much you'll spend on eating, drinking and entertainment once you reach your destination.

◯ Focus on rewarding activities that cost little or nothing – anything from walking in your local park, to going to free concerts, or visiting free art galleries and museums – so long as you enjoy it and it helps you concentrate on 'being' rather than 'having.'

Cut your food bills

Work out how much you can afford to spend on nourishing yourself and your family, and then aim to buy foods that form a healthy balanced diet (see Action 2, Eat fewer refined foods). Plan your meals for the week ahead, then make a list of the foods you need before you go shopping and stick to it. If you're on a tight budget, focus on meals made from cheap but nutritious ingredients, such as fruit and vegetables, pulses, potatoes, brown rice, wholemeal bread, wholewheat cereals, pasta and oats. Eggs, baked beans, tinned sardines and tuna are all economical sources of protein and other nutrients. Save money on basic foodstuffs by looking for the 'value' brands at major supermarkets, buying at cheaper superstores, or by buying in bulk; for example, by taking advantage of 'buy one get one free' or other special offers. Compare food prices at different supermarkets and shop from them by going to www.mysupermarket. co.uk. Choose foods that are priced down because they are close to their sell-by date. You can often buy fruit, vegetables and meats more cheaply at your local market, especially at the end of the day, or on a Saturday.

Make your own cheaper and healthier versions of ready meals by cooking extra portions of your favourite dishes and freezing them. Take a home-made sandwich, soup or salad, plus fruit and yoghurt, to work for lunch. Make your coffee at work rather than buying takeaway drinks from a cafe.

Grow your own vegetables; as well as saving you money they will be fresher and free from pesticides. You don't need a large garden or an allotment; you can grow a variety of vegetables, including potatoes, carrots, peas, tomatoes, beetroot and broad, French and runner beans in pots or containers. Use a deep pot or container. Put stones or broken pots in the bottom for drainage, then fill with compost before planting and watering (or use grow-bags as they tend to be cheaper).

Get the savings habit

A 2012 survey of 2,000 people for National Savings and Investments found that making regular savings boosted people's mood and gave them a sense of achievement; so squirrel away some of the money you've saved by being more frugal into a savings account. If you are a tax payer, an ISA will give you the best interest because it isn't taxed, otherwise check current rates on a money comparison site like www.moneysupermarket.com.

10. Cut work-related pressures

☐ **Prepare your clothes and packed lunch the night before** – do the same for your children if you have any.

☐ **Adjust your desk and chair so you can sit correctly** – with your feet flat on the floor, your pelvis slightly higher than your knees and your eyes in line with the top of your computer screen.

☐ **Keep a foliage plant on your desk** – its calming, air-purifying and humidifying effects will help to lower your blood pressure and stress levels, and boost your productivity.

☐ **Tidy your desk to help you focus on the task in hand** – put paperwork that needs to be acted on soon in your in-tray; file away paperwork you'll need later; and bin or recycle anything that is out of date or no longer needed.

☐ **Clear your computer desktop every month** – files and icons that you no longer use can be binned to free up memory space and help your computer (and you) to work more quickly and efficiently.

☐ **Write a to-do list at the end of your working day** – ready for the next day. Number tasks according to their urgency and importance, then complete them in that order, crossing them off your list as you go.

☐ **'Chunk' tasks** – if you have a few telephone calls to make, letters to write or emails to respond to, set aside a time to complete similar tasks together.

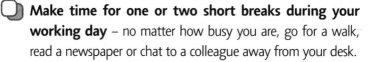

Avoid 'catching' stress – if a colleague is complaining about their work or personal life, try saying something positive or offer to help them. If they persist in being negative, take a break if possible or think positive thoughts to avoid adopting their mindset.

Make time for one or two short breaks during your working day – no matter how busy you are, go for a walk, read a newspaper or chat to a colleague away from your desk.

Get away from your desk every hour or two – to loosen muscles, boost blood flow and release endorphins; this will improve your productivity and mood and help prevent eye strain.

'Deskercise' if you don't have time to leave your desk – drop your head down towards your left shoulder, then your right; lift, then drop the shoulders, then circle backwards and forwards alternately; put your hands on the small of your back then arch your back, pushing your hips forwards and pulling your shoulders back; stretch your arms out in front of you then clench your fists and release.

Socialise

While too many interruptions from emails, phone calls, text messages and colleagues chatting can lead to work piling up, being sociable at work has been shown to reduce stress. So take five minutes for a chat, if you can, during your working day.

Switch off from work after hours – turn off your mobile phone and BlackBerry, and avoiding checking your emails. If you have to bring work equipment home, put it away out of sight and out of mind.

Confidence is key to a good career

In 2012, researchers at the University of California claimed that confidence was more important than skills, hard work or education when it comes to climbing the career ladder.

11. Change your attitude towards a stressful situation

Cognitive Behavioural Therapy (CBT) is a type of psychotherapy that aims to tackle negative thoughts and unhelpful behaviours that can lead to emotional problems, including stress and low self-confidence. According to cognitive theory, many of us form negative beliefs about ourselves through our experiences in childhood and early adulthood, e.g. being bullied at school, parents divorcing, failing an exam, etc., and these take root in our minds until they become second nature. Behavioural theory is based on the belief that behaviour is a learned response that is also a reaction to past experiences. CBT combines both types of theory.

According to CBT, an event or situation is only stressful if you believe it is, because your feelings aren't facts; they are just your perception of an event or situation and your ability to deal with it.

How you view and react to events in your life is down to the filters you view them through. These filters include your personality, values, beliefs and attitudes, which have been shaped by your genetics, upbringing, past experiences, lifestyle and culture. So it is possible to cut the amount of stress you feel about a situation simply by changing your perception of it and your ability to handle it.

Try this:

1. Write down the situation you feel stressed about, e.g. starting a new job.

2. Note down any negative thoughts you have about the situation and your ability to cope with it, e.g. 'I'm worried I won't be good enough at the job.'

3. Think of alternative, more positive ways of viewing the situation, e.g. 'The company must think I'm capable of doing the job, or they wouldn't have hired me'; 'I've succeeded in previous jobs, so I'm sure I can in this one.'

4. Think of helpful behaviours, e.g. 'I'll make a plan of how I'm going to tackle the job'; 'I'll ask questions if I'm unsure about anything.'

If you use this technique every time you face a testing situation, you will gradually find yourself viewing such events as a challenge rather than stressful, and feeling more confident in your ability to cope with whatever life throws at you.

12. Focus on the present

One of the most effective ways of reducing your stress levels is to practise living in the present, which is often referred to as mindfulness. Mindfulness involves paying attention to what is going on around you right now and helps to quieten the mind.

Dwelling on events from the past and worrying about what might happen in the future raises stress levels unnecessarily; and stress or worry can eat away at your self-confidence. The body's stress response cannot tell the difference between what is real and what is imagined, for example, if you worry about losing your job and being unable to pay your bills your body will release stress hormones, even if you keep your job. If you focus on the present instead, you'll probably find that many of your problems and worries disappear, and that you find it easier to concentrate on the task in hand and enjoy life as it unfolds, minute by minute.

Living in the present means you can focus your energies on dealing with real situations, rather than wasting it worrying about 'what ifs'. So, instead of agonising over what could go wrong at a forthcoming event, such as a meeting, job interview or exam, identify what you can do *now* to prepare for it (see Action 33, Plan to succeed), so that you feel more confident and in control.

Don't worry!

Studies suggest that 85 per cent of the things we worry about have a positive outcome.

13. Be mindful in everyday life

Good examples of being mindful in everyday life include participating in a sport or doing something in which you can 'lose yourself', like cooking a meal, painting a picture, knitting or sewing. Other examples of mindfulness include meditation (see actions 14–18), which requires you to focus on one thing, such as your breathing, an object, a thought or an image, and the Alexander Technique (see Action 41); this comprises a set of principles that help you improve your posture, and involves paying attention to how you are holding and moving your body, as well as identifying where you are carrying tension. Living in the present is a skill that can be learned; below are more examples of how you can practise mindfulness in the course of everyday life and focus on 'being' rather than 'doing'.

- **When you are out walking** – be aware of your breathing and how you are holding your body; focus on the feeling of your feet hitting the ground; then turn your attention to your surroundings; what can you see, hear, feel and smell? Notice the colours and shapes of your surroundings; listen to the sounds around you, for example, trees rustling in the breeze, birds chirping; feel the breeze or the warmth of the sun on your face; smell the cut grass or the scent of flowers.

- **When you are having a shower** – listen to the gushing sound of the water and feel the pressure and warmth of it melt away any tension in your muscles; smell the perfume of the soap or shower gel and shampoo you are using; notice the sensation of the sponge or washcloth on your skin and how refreshed and wide awake you feel afterwards.

When you are having a conversation – actively listen to the other person, concentrating on what they are saying, noticing their body language and the tone of their voice, instead of allowing your mind to wander. Don't worry if you find living in the present difficult initially; whenever your mind starts wandering just try to bring it back to the present. For more information on mindfulness take a look at the Mental Health Foundation's Be Mindful campaign at www.bemindful.co.uk.

Take time out to relax

With our ever faster pace of living it's more important than ever to take time out to relax. No matter how busy you are, try to fit in some 'me time' every day – even if it's just to go and have a long soak in the bath, sit and read a book or magazine for half an hour, or watch your favourite TV programme – anything that helps to take your mind off everyday worries and concerns will help to reduce your stress levels. If you prefer a more formal method of relaxation you could try meditation.

Meditate

Meditation is a form of mindfulness that involves focusing your mind on a specific activity, thought or object and disregarding any distractions. In the past many people have dismissed meditation as something that is practised by followers of religions like Zen Buddhism. However, in recent years it has become more mainstream, probably as a result of a growing body of clinical research which shows that meditating regularly promotes deep physical and mental relaxation, and combats the adverse effects of stress. As well as reducing stress levels, meditation can encourage positive thinking and an improved self-image, which is helpful for boosting self-confidence.

The following five actions are types of meditation: the first involves focusing on breathing deeply; the second involves focusing on breathing deeply while visualising a particular colour; the third involves picturing a relaxing retreat; the fourth involves focusing on a word or phrase (mantra); and the final one involves tensing then releasing your muscles, as you breathe in and out.

14. Breathe deeply

With each breath we take, oxygen is absorbed into the blood to produce the energy we need for all the different functions in our bodies. When we're stressed our breathing tends to be fast and shallow, which leads to a drop in the level of calming carbon dioxide in our bloodstream. This can make us even more stressed and cause muscular tension in the neck, shoulders and upper back. Slow, deep breathing slows the heart rate, increases production of calming alpha brainwaves, relaxes the muscles, relieves tension, and triggers the production of 'happy hormones' serotonin and dopamine. So the next time you're feeling stressed or worried – perhaps before a job interview or an exam – take control of your breathing.

1. Sit or lie comfortably.

2. Close your eyes and begin to focus on your breathing.

3. Inhale slowly and deeply through your nose to a count of five, allowing your stomach to expand. Hold for five seconds.

4. Exhale slowly for ten seconds, slowly drawing in your stomach.

5. Whenever a passing thought distracts you, simply return your attention to your breathing.

15. Practise colour breathing

Colour is all around us every day, both in the natural world and in man-made environments, influencing the way we think, feel and act without us even being aware of it. Colour is nature's own signalling system, and the way we respond to it is linked to our innate survival instinct; for example, in the natural world red often signifies danger and, as a result, when we see red our heart rate increases and we become more alert. Blue and green are the two main colours found in nature and they have been shown to calm and soothe. The effects may vary from one person to another but certain colours are generally linked to particular emotions, for example, yellow is associated with confidence, inner strength, optimism, willpower and determination, and red is thought to stimulate the mind and invoke courage and vitality.

Try this colour meditation next time you want to feel more confident and optimistic:

1. Follow the deep-breathing technique outlined in Action 14.

2. On each inhalation imagine you are breathing in the colour yellow and your body is filling up with it.

When you want to feel more alert and energetic try the same technique only imagine you're inhaling the colour red; to feel calmer try inhaling blue or green.

16. Visualise a relaxing retreat

Visualisation allows you to escape from everyday stresses and strains, and can be done whenever you have a few spare minutes. When you vividly imagine a pleasant scene your mind responds by releasing the same endorphins and other pleasure-giving chemicals it would if you were actually there.

1. Find a comfortable place to sit or lie and close your eyes.

2. Focus on breathing in and out slowly and deeply as in the previous exercises.

3. Now visualise a relaxing retreat, for example, a forest with tall green pine trees and a gently flowing stream, or a beach with white sand, blue skies, turquoise sea and lush palm trees.

4. Next, use each of your senses to vividly imagine every detail of your retreat; smell the aroma of the pine trees, hear the water gurgling, feel the warmth of the sun on your face and body, hear the crash and roar of the waves.

5. Enjoy the scene until you feel ready to return to reality.

6. Breathe in and out slowly and deeply. When you are ready, open your eyes.

17. Use a mantra

A mantra is a word or phrase that you use to induce a state of relaxation. A study at the Medical College of Wisconsin in 2012 involving 201 participants with an average age of 59 years, found that participants practising this form of meditation for 20 minutes twice daily had reduced stress and blood pressure levels and were 48 per cent less likely to have a heart attack, stroke or die from all causes, compared with participants who attended a health education class, over a period of over five years.

Try this:

1. Choose a word or phrase that suggests relaxation to you, such as: 'peace'; 'calm'; 'I am totally relaxed'; 'my muscles are relaxing'.

2. Sit quietly and shut your eyes.

3. Breathe in and out slowly, and deeply, as described in the previous exercises.

4. Repeat your mantra either out loud or in your head, on each out-breath.

5. If your mind wanders, simply bring it back to the mantra, repeating it with more emphasis.

18. Relax your muscles

Whenever you feel stressed you're likely to tense your muscles, which tends to make you feel even more stressed. When you release the tension from your muscles you naturally feel more relaxed. Try this muscle relaxation sequence before or after other meditations, or whenever you are feeling tense:

1. Inhale deeply through your nose, then tense your face muscles by clenching your jaw and screwing up your eyes tightly. Release the muscles in your face as you exhale through your mouth.

2. Take a deep breath in through your nose, then lift your shoulder muscles, tense for a few seconds and then allow them to fall, releasing the tension as you breathe out through your mouth.

3. Inhale deeply through your nose, then clench your fists and tighten the muscles in your arms, hold for a few seconds then release and exhale through your mouth.

4. Breathe in through your nose, tense the muscles in your buttocks and legs, hold, then relax them as you breathe out through your mouth.

5. Finally, breathe in through your nose, clench your toes and tense your feet, hold, then release them as you breathe out.

Speedy relaxer

Obviously, it isn't always convenient to follow this sequence when you are out and about. Below is a speedy muscle relaxation technique that you can practise discreetly any time, anywhere, without people noticing:

 Take a deep breath in through your nose, tightening up your shoulder and back muscles. Hold for five seconds.

 Breathe out through your mouth slowly, allowing your shoulders to fall and the muscles to relax.

 Imagine all of the tension drifting out of your body.

19. Sleep soundly

Stress is a major cause of poor sleep because it can affect levels of the sleep hormone melatonin. Poor sleep is also a major cause of stress; after just one night of poor-quality sleep we are less able to cope with pressure, and more likely to be suffering from low mood and irritability, have problems concentrating and remembering things, and more likely to succumb to infections and illness.

According to a survey of 5,300 people by Mental Health Matters in 2011, poor sleepers are also four times more likely to experience relationship problems and are twice as likely to suffer from fatigue. Lack of sleep is linked to weight gain too, as it lowers levels of the appetite-controlling hormone leptin. Also, research at the Karolinska Institute in Stockholm in 2010 suggested there is such a thing as 'beauty sleep'; a study found that volunteers were judged less attractive and healthy looking after a night with little or broken sleep compared with when they had a normal night's sleep. Feeling physically or mentally below par, being overweight or feeling unattractive can have a huge negative impact on your self-confidence, so making sure you sleep well is vital. Below are 20 top tips to help you sleep soundly:

1. **Get outdoors in daylight** – to halt the production of melatonin, the brain chemical that promotes sleep; this makes it easier for your body to release it at night, so you fall asleep more quickly and sleep more soundly. Blue light, which is light from a blue sky on a clear day, is believed to be the most beneficial.

2. **Eat foods rich in tryptophan** – an amino acid from which your body first produces mood-boosting serotonin and then the 'sleep' hormone melatonin. Tryptophan-rich foods include

chicken, turkey, bananas, dates, rice, oats, wholegrain breads, cereals and dairy foods, which also contain calming calcium, which is why a glass of milk at bedtime can help you sleep.

3. **Ensure you're neither hungry nor too full** – when you go to bed, as both can lead to wakefulness. Ideally, avoid eating a heavy meal later than two hours before bed. However, if you are hungry at bedtime, a light tryptophan-rich snack such as oatcakes and cheese, or a turkey or chicken sandwich, could help you to sleep more soundly.

4. **Avoid drinking coffee or cola, or eating chocolate after 3 p.m.** – it takes the body up to eight hours to break down the caffeine they contain and research at Tel Aviv University, Israel in 2002 found that as well as being a stimulant, caffeine reduces melatonin levels by half. While tea has about half the caffeine of coffee – around 50 mg per cup – it's best to avoid drinking it near bedtime if you have trouble sleeping. Instead, drink decaffeinated tea and coffee, dandelion or chicory coffee substitutes, redbush (rooibos) or herbal teas, all of which are caffeine-free (see Action 4, Cut down on caffeine).

5. **Avoid daytime naps and stick to a regular sleep schedule** – even if you've had a poor night's sleep and feel like a lie in; changing your sleeping patterns confuses your body clock and affects sleep quality, whereas going to bed and getting up at roughly the same time helps your body clock to function well and encourages sound sleep.

6. **Exercise to help you sleep** – it raises your body temperature and metabolism, which fall a few hours later, triggering sleepiness. Inactivity can cause restlessness and difficulty sleeping, however, avoid exercising in the three hours before you go to bed as exercise also increases brain activity, and your

body temperature could still be raised at bedtime, both of which could promote wakefulness.

7. **Unwind before bedtime** – develop your own evening routine that lets you 'put the day to bed'. This might include watching TV – if you find it helps you relax – but avoid anything that might prey on your mind later when you're trying to fall asleep and aim to switch the television off half an hour before bed at the latest. Many people find reading or listening to music helps them to relax.

8. **Dim the lights** – to encourage your body to release melatonin; a dimmer switch, lamp or candles are ideal for this.

9. **Soak in a warm bath before bed** – it raises your temperature, which then falls promoting sleep. The warmth can also help ease muscular and mental tension, especially if you add a few drops of relaxing essential oils like lavender, neroli or sandalwood.

10. **Avoid drinking alcohol at bedtime** – it might help you relax and drop off more quickly, but it can disrupt sleep patterns, so that you have less deep sleep. It is also a diuretic, so you are more likely to make trips to the toilet during the night. However, one glass of red wine made from grape skins that are especially rich in melatonin – such as Cabernet Sauvignon, Merlot or Chianti – two or three hours before bed could help you sleep.

11. **Make sure your bedroom is cool and inviting** – your brain tries to lower your body temperature at night to slow down your metabolism and promote sleep; around 18°C is ideal. Make your bedroom a comfortable retreat with fresh bedding and soft lighting to make bedtime a pleasure. Decorate the room in colours you find relaxing, for most people this will be neutral and pastel shades.

12. **Hang dark, heavy curtains, or black-out blinds, or wear an eye mask** – to block out the light. Darkness stimulates the pineal gland in the brain to produce melatonin.

13. **Check your mattress gives you the right level of support** – lie on your back then slip a hand under your lower back. There should be just enough space to fit your hand in the gap between your back and the mattress. If you can't, the mattress is too soft for you. A bed board under the mattress might help. If the gap is bigger than this, the mattress is too hard.

14. **Pick a pillow that aligns your spine with your neck** – the best pillow thickness for you depends on the width of your shoulders; if you have narrow shoulders choose a flatter pillow, if you are broad-shouldered, you might need two pillows. Memory foam pillows are another good choice, as they mould to your shape to support your head and neck. You can also buy pillows shaped to suit how you sleep, i.e. on your back, side or stomach.

15. **Banish TVs, computers, iPads and mobile phones** – to help your brain associate your bedroom with sleep and sex only. Watching TV or using a computer or other technology last thing at night can over-stimulate your brain, making it hard to switch off and get to sleep; processing huge amounts of information from these devices means we get less of the deep restorative sleep we need to feel refreshed. Screens also give off bright light, which can hamper melatonin production.

16. **Reduce noise** – from traffic or your partner's snoring by wearing earplugs. Research shows that nearly a quarter of insomniacs blame noise for their lack of sleep.

17. **Clear your mind of worries** – about problems or events happening the next day by jotting down your concerns or a plan for the day ahead before bed.

18. **Only go to bed when you feel sleepy** – if you don't drop off within about 20 minutes, get up and do something you find relaxing, like reading or listening to soothing music. Only return to bed when you feel drowsy to help your brain associate your bed with sleep.

19. **If you still feel tense when your head hits the pillow** – try visualising a relaxing retreat or relaxing your muscles as outlined in Actions 16 and 18.

20. **If you can't sleep try not to worry about it** – this will only make it harder to drop off – focus instead on getting comfortable and relaxed – remember resting is the next best thing to sleep. With a more relaxed outlook you may even find yourself sleeping better!

Avoid dwelling on problems during the night

If you wake during the night and start mulling over problems, try telling yourself firmly: 'You can't do anything about this right now, so go to sleep and deal with it tomorrow.'

Chapter 4

Think Yourself Confident

In this chapter we look at how your thoughts affect your confidence. It is estimated that we have around 50,000 thoughts every day. If your thoughts about yourself and your experiences are mainly positive you are likely to be confident and self-assured; if you tend to think about yourself critically you are more likely to lack self-confidence; perfectionism and comparing yourself with other people are often responsible for these negative thought patterns.

If you are confident about yourself and your abilities you are more likely to succeed in life and, as a result, think well of yourself. If you have low self-confidence you may not achieve your full potential and this will reinforce the negative thoughts and beliefs you have about yourself. In other words, your thoughts affect your confidence, which in turn affects your performance, which then comes full circle to affect your thoughts again. For example, if you think: 'I can't do presentations', you are likely to lack confidence when giving a presentation, which means you are more likely to perform badly, thus backing up your belief that you can't do presentations.

This chapter explains why you should avoid the pursuit of perfectionism, as well as how to challenge any negative thoughts and beliefs you have about yourself and replace them with more realistic and positive ones, so that you develop a higher opinion of yourself and, as a result, become more confident and self-assured.

20. Avoid comparing yourself with others

Why compare yourself with others? No one in the entire world can do a better job of being you than you.
Anonymous

One of the personality traits that can trigger negative thoughts and beliefs about yourself is perfectionism and comparing yourself unfavourably with other people. The media plays a big part in many people's tendency to put themselves down because they distort our view of what is 'normal' with a constant stream of images of beautiful people with high-flying careers, dressed in designer clothes, and living in large pristine houses with all the latest gadgets and technology, and driving top-of-the range cars. When people find that they can't match these impossible ideals they begin to feel that they don't quite measure up, which chips away at their self-confidence.

The problem is these so-called perfect lives are an illusion; in reality the models and celebrities on TV and in the newspapers only look that way after hours spent in make-up and with extensive airbrushing; the person with the high-flying career and lifestyle to match may be stressed and unhappy trying to hang on to them; and A-list celebrities might feel under a lot of pressure to remain at the top of their game. Whilst it's good to have goals – achieving them will help you to develop your skills and talents and build your confidence in your abilities – they need to be realistic and reflect your wants and needs, not some artificially constructed ideal.

So, instead of putting yourself down because your body, clothes, lifestyle or achievements aren't as good as someone else's, recognise that your shape, personality, talents, skills and experiences are unique to you, and no one is perfect; everyone has both positive and negative traits and strengths and weaknesses.

Try this: Instead of thinking 'I want to be like her/him', think: 'I want to be the best I can be.'

To break the negative thought – poor performance – lack of confidence cycle you need to challenge the negative thoughts and beliefs you have about yourself and replace them with more positive, but realistic ones. Remember your thoughts aren't facts; they are simply your perception of the truth.

21. Challenge your confidence-sapping thoughts

Self-critical thinking patterns develop in response to events and experiences throughout your life. For example, if your parents or teachers criticised you, you were bullied at school, you failed an exam, or a loved one ended a relationship, you might have reacted with thoughts like: 'I'm not good enough'; 'Other people don't like me'; 'I'm a failure'; I'm unlovable'. Once these critical thoughts take hold they become automatic and sap your confidence. However, it is possible to overcome your inner critic by challenging the faulty reasoning behind your self-critical thoughts and replacing them with more balanced, positive ones.

Try this:
1. For a week record all of your negative and self-critical thoughts and beliefs.

2. At the end of the week select up to five self-critical thoughts or beliefs.

3. Now challenge each one by identifying the faulty logic behind it, questioning it and creating more balanced thoughts and beliefs.

Below are some of the most common types of faulty reasoning, with examples of the types of thoughts they can lead to and how these can affect your confidence, as well as how to challenge and replace them with alternative, positive beliefs.

Mislabelling
What it is: this is where you rate yourself on the basis of one negative event.
Example: You tell yourself 'I'm a failure' after failing one exam.
Effect on confidence: You lack confidence when sitting any test or exam in the future.
How to challenge: Remind yourself that you are human and therefore sometimes get things wrong, but that doesn't make you a failure.
New thought/belief: 'I've passed exams in the past'; 'I am a success'.

Catastrophising
What it is: This is where you turn a minor event into a major one.
Example: You make a mistake at work and start thinking 'I'm hopeless at my job'.
Effect on confidence: You doubt your ability to do your job and think you are about to be dismissed.
How to challenge: Put things into perspective by telling yourself it's only one mistake and you wouldn't have held down your job if you weren't capable of doing it.
New thought/belief: 'Everyone makes mistakes and mine was just a small one'; 'I am competent at my job'.

'All or nothing' thinking
What it is: This is where you have an extreme view of yourself, i.e. you are good or bad at something, a success or a failure.
Example: You stopped smoking a month ago but had one cigarette on a night out so you tell yourself 'I've ruined everything'.

Effect on confidence: You decide you lack the commitment to quit and start smoking again.

How to challenge: Tell yourself that some events fall somewhere in between success and failure.

New thought/belief: 'I had a temporary setback, but I can still give up smoking'; 'I am still a non-smoker'.

Mind-reading

What it is: This is where you guess what other people are thinking about you.

Example: One of your colleagues at work is abrupt with you so you think: 'They don't like me. There must be something wrong with me.'

Effect on confidence: You worry that you might have said or done something to upset your colleague and feel uncomfortable about working with them.

How to challenge: Remind yourself that you can't possibly know what someone else is thinking. Think of alternative explanations for your colleague's behaviour, for example they may have been tired or hungry, or have personal problems. Remind yourself that you get on well with other colleagues and have lots of friends.

New thought/belief: 'I have lots of friends'; 'I am well-liked'.

Fortune-telling

What it is: This is where you make negative predictions about a future event.

Example: You feel apprehensive about making a presentation and tell yourself 'I'm going to mess this up'.

Effect on confidence: Your confidence in your ability to deliver the presentation nosedives and you start to believe that you won't be able to do it.

How to challenge: Tell yourself that you can't predict the future. Think about similar events in the past where you thought you would do badly but they turned out well. Tackle your fears by preparing thoroughly for the presentation.

New thought/belief: 'I can't predict the future, but I can prepare well and do my best'; 'I am capable of delivering a great presentation'.

Ignoring the positive
What it is: This is where your lack of confidence colours your perception of positive feedback or events.

Example: You are complimented on your performance at work by your boss, but dismiss the positive feedback by telling yourself: 'They probably say that to everyone. I'm nothing special.'

Effect on confidence: You keep your negative beliefs about yourself going.

How to challenge: Take on board the positive feedback instead of dismissing it. Vow to accept all compliments in the future.

New thought/belief: 'I'm doing well at work'; 'I'm competent and worthy'.

Now that you have the tools to challenge your negative thoughts, make sure you keep using them whenever the need arises; eventually you should find that whenever an event triggers self-doubts and put-downs you will automatically identify your thinking errors and look for alternative, more positive, thoughts and beliefs.

Chapter 5

Exude Confidence

As we discussed at the beginning of this book, confidence is not only about belief in yourself and your abilities; it's also about being able to project this inner certainty. Studies show that when you adopt the body language, voice and vocabulary of a confident person you feel more confident. This is because holding yourself well prompts the body to release confidence-boosting chemicals, and speaking calmly, with positive words, also makes you feel more self-assured. Also, when you project yourself well people respond to you more positively, which again improves confidence. This chapter offers techniques to help you present yourself in a way that reflects your inner-confidence and increases it.

Part of being confident is being able to ask for what you want, say what you really feel and say 'no' to the things you don't want to do without feeling guilty, and without upsetting other people; the last section in the chapter covers assertiveness skills to help you do this.

22. Adopt confident body language

Body language is about how we hold our bodies and the gestures we make. We may not be aware of it most of the time, but our body language reveals how we are feeling and what we are thinking, it plays a huge part in how we communicate with others and how they perceive us. For example, a depressed person who is lacking in confidence tends to hunch their shoulders and look down at the ground, whereas someone who is happy and self-assured is more likely to stand tall and look straight ahead. When we are worried we tend to frown; when we are feeling vulnerable we may cross our arms as if to protect ourselves; when we are feeling impatient we might drum our fingers as if we are trying to speed things up.

Research suggests that we can also manipulate our body language to change the way we feel. In 2010 a study at Harvard and Columbia universities noted an increase in testosterone levels and a fall in stress hormone levels among participants who adopted confident 'power' poses, i.e. they took up more space by using 'open' body language. They also behaved more confidently and said they felt more powerful than participants who adopted 'low power poses', i.e. they took up less space by crossing their arms and legs. The testosterone levels of the 'low power' posture participants fell and their stress hormone levels went up. Higher testosterone levels are associated with assertiveness and energy. The researchers concluded that people can feel more confident and perform better in challenging situations like going for a job interview or speaking in public simply by adopting a confident stance.

Use the power pose
Try it for yourself; next time your confidence needs a quick boost try adopting a power pose:

1. Sit or stand tall, looking straight ahead.

2. Take a deep breath and imagine that you are inflating and taking up more space.

3. Use open body language; take a wide stance with both feet planted firmly on the floor.

4. Make sure your arms, legs, knees and feet are open (not crossed).

5. Relax your shoulders and let your arms hang loosely at your sides.

6. Use open gestures, for example hold your hands apart and open rather than clasped.

For more information about improving your posture in general see Action 41, Perfect your posture with the Alexander Technique.

Smile!

Studies show that when we smile the brain releases feel-good endorphins, so we project a more relaxed and confident image. As a result other people react more positively to us, which also boosts confidence.

23. Find your confident 'chocolate voice'

We all have two types of voice; one is a high-pitched, squeaky voice that originates in the throat or nose and suggests nervousness and a lack of confidence; the other is a deeper, calmer voice that comes from the stomach and projects confidence, self-assuredness and authority.

To find your confident voice imagine you are eating some delicious chocolate (or something else you love the taste of); take a deep breath in, allowing your stomach to expand, hold it for a second and then breathe out from your stomach and make an 'mmmmm' sound as though you are tasting the chocolate. If you are doing it correctly your voice should vibrate. Use this technique whenever you are in a situation where you have to speak in public and you are feeling nervous, ill at ease or lacking in confidence.

24. Choose your words carefully

Words conjure up images and feelings, so just like your thoughts, what you say affects how you feel and act. For example, if you were to say: 'The maths exam is going to be really hard,' you would probably feel daunted and dispirited. If instead you said something like: 'The maths exam is going to be a challenge,' you would be more likely to feel positive, motivated and confident about doing it. Or if you were to say: 'I'm terrified about my job interview tomorrow,' you probably would feel terrified, and again this would have a negative impact on your confidence and performance.

On the other hand, if you said: 'I'm excited about my job interview tomorrow,' you would be more likely to feel positive and motivated to do your best. So choose your words carefully, especially before an important event.

Below are more examples of the power of changing negative statements into positive, confidence-boosting ones.

'I have to' or **'I must'** – which immediately put you on your guard and de-motivate you. If you said **'I choose to'** or **'I want to'** instead you would feel much more inspired and empowered.

'Life's a struggle' – suggests life is something to be endured, whereas **'Life's an adventure'** is more motivating and encouraging.

'If only I had' – implies regret, whereas **'Next time I will'** promotes the idea that you can learn from past mistakes and do better next time.

25. Learn the rules of assertion

When your confidence is low it's likely that you:

1. Avoid saying what you really want, feel or need.

2. Agree with other people's opinions to avoid hurting, offending or upsetting them, or to gain their approval.

3. Allow people to talk you into doing things you don't really want to do.

You may have started acting passively because your confidence in your ability to stand up for yourself has been eroded as a result of past experiences, such as being criticised by parents or teachers, or other pupils bullying or making fun of you at school. When you fail to assert yourself you may feel less anxious or guilty in the short term, but in the long term your self-confidence will remain low, and bottling up your feelings may cause stress and depression.

Learning how to be more assertive will enable you to say what you want, feel and need, and stand up for your rights confidently and calmly, without being aggressive or hurting other people's feelings. This will encourage others to treat you with respect, which will boost your confidence.

To give you some idea of what being assertive means, below is a list of rules of assertion; believing that you have these rights indicates strong self-worth.

The rules of assertion

I have the right to:

1. Express my feelings, beliefs and opinions.

2. Ask for what I want.

3. Say 'no'.

4. Change my mind.

5. Be listened to.

6. Recognise my individual needs.

7. Set my own priorities.

8. Take pride in my successes.

9. Decline responsibility for other adults' actions.

10. Make mistakes.

Say what you want, feel and need

The following tactics will help you to express your feelings and opinions, and stay in control of your life, doing things because you want to, rather than to please other people.

○ Pick the right time and place to talk, i.e. when you can talk in private and not when the other person appears to be busy or tired.

○ Make eye contact but don't stare, as the other person may find this intimidating.

○ Speak calmly, clearly and firmly, but without raising your voice.

○ Plan exactly what you want to say before you start speaking.

○ Aim to be concise and to the point, rather than rambling.

○ Use the word 'I' to show that you are taking responsibility for your own thoughts, feelings and behaviour rather than 'we', 'you' or 'it'. So instead of saying 'You hurt my feelings when you…' try something like 'I feel hurt when you…' – this is less accusatory and antagonistic to the other person.

○ When you can choose whether or not to do something, say 'I am not' or 'I don't want to' instead of 'I can't' to reflect that you've made an active decision, rather than making it sound as though something, or someone, has stopped you. Use 'I want to' instead of 'I have to', and 'I could', rather than 'I should', to show you have a choice. For example: 'I'm not going out tonight', or 'I don't want to go out tonight,' instead of 'I can't go out tonight'.

If you think the other person isn't listening to what you are saying, use the 'broken-record' technique: think of what you want to say, then keep repeating it, stating what you feel, want or need clearly and calmly, until the other person shows they have taken your comments on board. Respond to legitimate points raised by the other person, but ignore irrelevant arguments or criticisms. Avoid getting irritated, loud or angry, as you could come across as being aggressive. Using the aforementioned example, the conversation might go like this:

Susan: 'Do you want to go out for a meal tonight?'
Mary: 'I don't want to. I'm tired after being at work all week.'
Susan: 'We could just pop out for a couple of hours.'
Mary: 'I don't want to. I'm tired after being at work all week.'
Susan: 'You'd enjoy it when you get there.'
Mary: 'I don't want to. I'm tired after being at work all week.'
Susan: 'OK, I'll ask someone else.'

When making a request, specify what you want using positive, assertive words. For example, if you want to ask someone to help with the household chores you might say: 'I'd really appreciate it if you could empty the dishwasher.'

Give the other person the opportunity to respond to your comments or requests.

When you have more than one point to make, pause before the next one, so that the other person has a chance to digest each piece of information.

When refusing a request, state why without apologising. For example: 'I'm not coming to see you today, because I've been really busy at work all week and want to relax at home.'

If you disagree with someone, say so using the word 'I'. Explain why you disagree, but acknowledge the other person's right to have an opposing viewpoint. For example: 'I don't think I'm being selfish by wanting to stay at home today, but I know you look forward to my visits so I can understand why you think that.'

Once you start acting more assertively you should find that people respect you more for being honest and open with them and this will in turn boost your confidence. It is also better for your mental and physical wellbeing, and therefore your confidence, if you express how you feel, rather than bottling up negative emotions. Furthermore, it is beneficial for your relationships, as sometimes people bottle things up until they reach breaking point and then end up saying things they regret, or get really upset.

Chapter 6

Identify and Develop Your Strengths and Talents

Confidence comes from using your strengths and doing the things you are naturally good at and enjoy, because when you do something well you increase your belief in your abilities. In this chapter you will find exercises to help you recognise your natural abilities and identify how you can use them in everyday life.

26. Identify and play to your strengths

Your strengths are your positive character traits. Identifying your personal strengths will help to boost your confidence in two ways; firstly it will help you to develop a more positive view of yourself, and secondly it will help you to make choices in life that play to your strengths, so that you are more likely to be successful and confident. Many of the strengths listed on the next pages are needed for strong self-confidence and success in life – in particular courage, optimism and persistence.

Try this: Note down your major life events and achievements, then next to each one jot down the personal strengths you think you showed and drew upon in each situation.

The list below might give you some ideas:

 Kindness

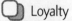 Empathy

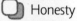 Loyalty

 Honesty

 Fairness

 Open-mindedness

 Forgiveness

 Gratitiude

 Love of learning

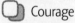 Communication

 Courage

Optimism

Persistence

Self-discipline

☐ Creativity

☐ Curiosity

☐ Modesty

☐ Vitality

☐ Leadership

☐ Organisation

☐ Teamwork

Play to your strengths

Next ask: Do I play to my personal strengths at work and at home? If your answer is 'no', identify ways you could make more use of your strengths. For example, if you love learning new things, ask to undertake some ongoing training to help you develop your skills and progress in your job; alternatively you could enrol on a course in something you'd love to learn about, for example, a foreign language, local history, floristry, interior design – the list is endless. Learning something new broadens your horizons and with every new skill you acquire your confidence will grow. If you're a good organiser, perhaps you could take on an organisational role at home, for example managing the household budget, arranging holidays, writing the shopping list, planning weekly menus, etc. Maybe you could use your organisational skills at work by setting and meeting deadlines, initiating ideas, delegating tasks and arranging meetings, or by finding a job that requires these sorts of skills.

If you have difficulty in recognising your strengths, ask your partner, a family member or a friend you trust what positive qualities they have noticed in you.

27. Recognise and use your talents

Your talents are the tasks and activities you have a natural aptitude for. The people who have got to the top of their chosen fields have done so by using and developing their innate talents and becoming the best they can at what they do. Good examples include: Michael McIntyre, Bradley Wiggins, Mick Jagger, Keira Knightley and Delia Smith.

Identifying, using and developing your innate abilities allows you to shine, so you can achieve more and be successful, which in turn creates confidence.

Everyone has at least one skill they can excel at. Perhaps you are unusually good at mental arithmetic, writing, languages, public speaking, teaching, cookery, gardening, interior design, singing or acting? Or maybe your skills lie in sports, playing a musical instrument, or arts and crafts? If you do the things you are really good at in life you are more likely to reach your full potential and develop strong self-confidence as a result.

When I was a college tutor delivering a course to help mature adults develop their confidence before starting an access to higher education course, I asked my students to list ten things they were good at. Several were women who had been out of education and employment for several years whilst raising a family; some of them completed the task with relative ease, whilst others struggled to think of more than a couple. Then as soon as I asked them if they had successfully raised children, cooked meals, cleaned and decorated their homes, organised the family finances and holidays, etc. it dawned on them that they were good at many things.

Now list your top ten talents:

1. ....

2. ....

3. ....

4. ....

5. ....

6. ....

7. ....

8. ....

9. ....

10. ....

If you find it difficult, try this:

1. Write down tasks you do well without having to try too hard. The tasks you learn quickly and can do almost effortlessly are the ones you have an innate talent for.

2. Now note down your passions. What do you really love to do? What excites and inspires you?

3. Finally, study both lists and pick out any common activities; these are the areas you are most likely to excel in and gain

self-fulfilment from. Now that you know where your natural abilities lie, check whether you are using and developing them, either at work or at home.

If you feel that you aren't using and developing your talents, start looking for ways in which you could. For example, if you are naturally good with animals you might run a dog-walking service in your spare time. If you love making jams and chutneys maybe you could make and sell them as a sideline. Developing your skills and making money at the same time is a great way of increasing your confidence as well as your bank balance!

These might sound like obvious things to do, but it's surprising how many people spend their lives doing jobs they don't particularly enjoy and waste their spare time watching TV or doing chores, when they could be doing the things they have a passion for and could achieve excellence in. If you are naturally talented at something, you might eventually find a way to develop it from a hobby or sideline into a full-time career or business. For example, the Duchess of Cambridge's mother Carole started her mail-order company, Party Pieces, in the garden shed! You will find advice on setting and achieving goals to help you improve your skills, achieve your dreams and increase your confidence in Chapter 8.

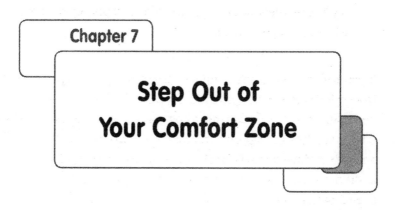

Chapter 7

Step Out of
Your Comfort Zone

Your comfort zone is basically all of the situations in which you feel confident and 'at home'; for example, doing the job you've done for a long time, socialising with a group of people you know well or living in a place you've lived all your life. In this chapter we are going to examine why we have all have comfort zones and the benefits of stepping outside of them. We'll also look at how fear keeps us stuck in our comfort zone and how we can overcome it. What most people are afraid of is taking risks – the risk of uncertainty, of making mistakes, of failure – so we look at how you can change your attitude towards risks, so that you view them as opportunities.

28. Discover the benefits of stepping out of your comfort zone

Stepping out of your comfort zone, for example, starting a new job, going to a party where you don't know anyone or moving to another part of the country, can be frightening, but whenever you do so your confidence grows.

Confident people also have comfort zones, but the difference between them and people lacking in confidence is that they are willing to take risks and try new things despite their fears. Confidence comes from taking action, not from inaction; each time you succeed in doing something you fear your comfort zone will expand. If you drive, think of your first driving lesson – you were probably terrified at the thought of driving 100 metres – but as you gradually improved your skills your confidence grew and now you could probably drive 100 miles without worrying.

If you lack confidence you may find yourself 'stuck' in a situation you are unhappy with – such as being in a relationship that is no longer working, spending hours travelling to work on the bus or train because you fear learning to drive, or doing a job you dislike or find unfulfilling – because you are too afraid to take the first step towards changing your life.

29. Be prepared to take a risk

Confidence is a funny thing. You go out and do the thing you're most terrified of, and the confidence comes afterwards.
Christopher Kaminski

Often it is not the fear of the actual situation that keeps us stuck in our comfort zone; it's usually a fear of the unknown, a fear of failure or a fear of making a mistake.

Fear of the unknown – staying in an unhappy relationship because you fear being alone and never meeting anyone else.

Fear of failure – fear of failing to achieve your goal; for example, taking driving lessons then failing your test.

 Fear of making a mistake – for example, fear that if you apply for a new job and you are successful you might not like it, or you may not be able to do it and be asked to leave. Then you would have to face the uncertainty of unemployment and end up feeling that you'd made a mistake and wishing you had stayed put.

What all of these scenarios involve is taking a risk. Risking being alone, risking failing your driving test, risking making a mistake by leaving your job; but the truth is nothing in life is certain; everything we do in life involves risks. If you are in an unhappy relationship there's a risk your partner might leave you first; if you don't try to learn to drive there's a risk you could limit your horizons; your current job could come to an end if the company folds.

Furthermore, if you let your fears stop you from taking action and stay in the 'safety' of your comfort zone you could miss out on countless opportunities. To take the three aforementioned examples; if you leave an unhappy relationship you are opening up the opportunity to start a new, happy one. If you start taking driving lessons you may find that you have a natural aptitude and pass your test first time. If you go for the new job you might love it and even if you don't it might lead to other opportunities.

Try this:
When you want to try something new, instead of viewing it as a risk look at it as an opportunity to expand your horizons; even if it goes wrong you will have learned from the experience.

The next action is a technique you can use to help you stretch the boundaries of your comfort zone.

30. Project past positive emotions

If you are worried about a forthcoming event where you need to perform well, for example, a job interview, an exam or a driving test, try tapping into the positive emotions you felt when you did something well in the past.

Think of your past successes and achievements. For example, winning a race at school sports day; passing an exam with flying colours; getting a job you really wanted; passing your driving test; or achieving a degree. Now think back to the positive emotions you felt at the time, for example, elation, pride, competence and confidence. Next, visualise yourself at the forthcoming event where you want to feel confident and be successful. As you picture the scene feel the positive emotions you felt when you looked back. Do this over and over again before the event; each time you do this you are preparing yourself mentally to feel confident and be successful by projecting the positive emotions you felt in the past onto the new event. The past achievement you choose to focus on doesn't have to be similar to the forthcoming one, because it is the emotion that you felt that you are using.

In the next chapter we look at how you can acknowledge past successes and build on them by setting goals. We also look at how to use visualisations in more detail, along with positive statements called affirmations. Using these techniques enables you to mentally practise the things you fear, so that when you come to do them you will feel 'safe' rather than threatened.

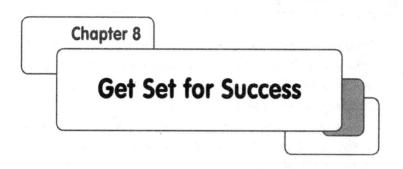

Chapter 8

Get Set for Success

Now that you have identified your strengths and talents, you are ready to set goals that enable you to develop them. Working towards meaningful goals will give you a sense of purpose; achieving them will give you a sense of pride and increase your overall feelings of competence and confidence.

This chapter aims to help you choose specific goals that matter to you, so that you feel motivated to achieve them by taking appropriate action. First of all you will be encouraged to acknowledge your past successes; when you do this you are reinforcing your belief in your abilities and reminding yourself that you have achieved your goals in the past, therefore you can do so again. You will discover how to set specific, measurable, ambitious, realistic and timed (SMART) goals and how to break them down into achievable initial steps and regular success habits (the long-term daily/weekly/monthly actions you need to take), so that you can track and acknowledge your progress and greatly improve your chances of success. We all know that in real life it isn't always easy to stick to our plans, no matter how determined we are, so there is a section on identifying possible obstacles and creating solutions before you begin working towards your goals. You'll also learn how to tap into the power of your subconscious mind to help achieve your goals by creating and using effective affirmations.

31. Acknowledge past successes

This is a sure-fire way to boost your confidence and motivate yourself to do well in the future. In the course of day-to-day living it's easy to forget the things you have done well in the past; focusing on your past successes helps to build your confidence in your abilities, especially if it's taken a knock.

Try this: List your top ten successes below.

1. ....

2. ....

3. ....

4. ....

5. ....

6. ....

7. ....

8. ....

9. ....

10. ....

If you're struggling to think of ten things, you're not alone; many of my past students couldn't think of any at first. However, when they cast their minds back over their lives in more detail they soon realised many of the successes they had forgotten about, or disregarded, were achievements they could be proud of. Past successes they identified that might help you think of your own include: 'Completing the Duke of Edinburgh's Silver Award'; 'Gaining my 25-metre swimming award'; 'Winning a local drawing competition'; 'Winning a football trophy'; 'Passing all of my GCSEs'; 'Passing my driving test'; and 'Bringing up my children well on my own'. Now give yourself a pat on the back for what you have achieved in the past and, whenever you doubt your ability to achieve your goals, return to your list of successes, and if you can, add some more!

32. Choose goals that excite and inspire you

What do you want to be, achieve and have? Choose goals that you feel passionate about and that use and develop the strengths and talents you identified in Chapter 6. Think about each area of your life, for example family, relationship, friendships, social life, career, finance, health and fitness, spirituality, fun and adventure, and write down how you would like them to be in your dream life.

Don't plan to do something to please someone else, or because you feel that you should; choose something that you really want to do, that inspires and excites you, then you'll have the motivation to persevere until you achieve your goal.

Set SMART goals
To increase your chances of success a goal should be:
Specific – define exactly what you want to achieve.
Measurable – can be measured, so that you will know when you have reached it.
Ambitious – your goal should stretch your abilities.
Realistic – you should believe you can achieve it.
Timed – set a deadline, but be prepared to extend it if you have to.

The most important thing is that you keep on working towards your target until you reach it.

Examples:
Career
Vague goal: 'To change my job.'
SMART goal: 'To retrain as a teaching assistant by the end of next June.'

Stopping smoking
Vague goal: 'To stop smoking.'
SMART goal: 'To stop smoking by the end of next month.'

33. Plan to succeed

If you fail to plan, you are planning to fail!
Benjamin Franklin

Once you have identified your goal you now need to create a plan outlining why you want to achieve it, the benefits of achieving it and how you will do it, including the initial steps you will need to take and the habits you will need to adopt to be successful. Writing down your motivation for and the benefits of achieving your goal will help you to commit to it. Planning the actions you will need to take will help you to break your goal down into manageable steps and enable you to track your progress.

Key points to consider:
Why do you want it?
Why do you want to achieve your goal? What benefits will you enjoy when you have reached your aim? These benefits will be your reward for all the hard work you put in, and will help to keep you going when you face disappointments and setbacks.

How will you do it?

To achieve anything in life you have to take action. The most effective way to reach any goal is to break it down into easy, attainable steps. With most goals there will be a few initial steps that you will need to take to set you off on the road towards achieving it. In your goal plan you will list these steps and record when you achieve each one; this will boost your confidence and encourage you to keep going.

Examples:

Goal: To retrain as a teaching assistant by the end of next June.
First steps:

1. Ring local schools to ask if I can volunteer.

2. Find out about local teaching assistant courses.

3. Enrol on a teaching assistant course.

Goal: To stop smoking by the end of next month.
First steps:

1. Make an appointment with my GP to find out what support is available from the NHS.

2. Discuss my options with an adviser and select the programme that suits me best.

3. Tell my family and friends when I intend to stop smoking and ask for their support.

34. Identify your success habits

Most goals are achieved and maintained by taking new long-term actions that you repeat daily/weekly/monthly until they become a habit that you do without thinking. Top Olympic athletes didn't achieve a gold medal after a week's intense training; they would have trained day in, day out, month in, month out, until it became automatic. Research suggests that the key to winning in any athletic sport is to create a training routine and stick to it, no matter what. The same applies to achieving any goal. Taking the above examples of finding a new job and stopping smoking: you are more likely to find a new job if you search for one every day, and you are more likely to stop smoking if you develop a new daily routine that doesn't involve smoking, and stick to it. When it comes to achieving goals it is the little things you do every day/week/month that bring success, so work out which new habits you would need to adopt in order to reach your goal.

Examples:
Goal: To retrain as a teaching assistant by the end of next June.
Daily success habits:
1. Volunteer at a local school.
2. Complete a piece of coursework.

Weekly success habits:
1. Attend a teaching assistant course.
2. Plan a weekly study timetable.

Monthly success habits:
1. Check that I am up to date with coursework.
2. Reward myself for sticking to my study timetable with a small treat.

Goal: To stop smoking by the end of next month.
Daily success habits:
1. Chew some sugar-free gum or suck a mint whenever I get the urge to smoke.

2. Put the money I would have spent on cigarettes into a jar.

3. Mark each day since I last had a cigarette on a calendar.

Weekly success habits:
1. Tell myself I've done well to stop smoking.

2. Buy myself a small treat with some of the money I've saved, e.g. a magazine, a book or a new perfume/aftershave.

Monthly success habits:
1. Count the money I've saved in my jar and put it in my bank account.

2. Make a list of health benefits I've noticed; for example, being able to walk faster without wheezing, enjoying my food more because I can smell and taste it better.

35. Overcome obstacles

You might now be thinking: 'All of this sounds great and looks good on paper but things are never that easy in real life are they? What if I can't stick to my plans for some reason? What will I do then – just give up?'

Achieving a goal requires resilience. Resilience is basically the ability to bounce back after obstacles or setbacks, and take positive action to resolve issues, rather than simply giving up and abandoning your goal. The best way to overcome obstacles is to identify some you might have to deal with and possible solutions before you begin, that way you can prevent, or at least be prepared for, things that might go wrong.

Bear in mind most goals aren't achieved overnight – they are usually the result of sticking to regular habits – so falling by the wayside now and again won't stop you from reaching your goal in the long term, so long as you return to your regular success habits as soon as you can. Instead of putting yourself down, think positively. For example: 'I've done really well to get this far. One mistake or setback isn't going to stop me from succeeding.'

Example:
Goal: To stop smoking by the end of next month.
Obstacles:

1. Some of my friends smoke.

2. I always feel tempted to smoke when I feel stressed.

Solutions

1. Avoid socialising with friends who are smokers for the first few weeks of giving up smoking.

2. Practise deep breathing whenever I feel stressed.

36. Create and use positive affirmations

In Chapter 4 we looked at how you can boost your confidence by challenging the negative thoughts and beliefs you have about yourself. An affirmation works in a similar way; it is a positive written statement about yourself that you repeat again and again until your subconscious mind believes it is true and you start behaving accordingly.

An effective affirmation should be:

1. **Personal** – because you can only change your own behaviour, no one else's, so always include the word 'I'.

2. **Positive** – how you think affects how you act, so state what you want to achieve, rather than what you don't.

3. **Present tense** – as if it is happening now.

4. **Achievement oriented** – use phrases like 'I have', 'I do', 'I am', 'I can'.

5. **Emotional** – describing how you will feel when you reach your goal will make it feel more real, e.g. 'confident', 'happy', 'relaxed', 'energetic'.

6. **Realistic** – is it achievable?

So, if your goal is 'to stop smoking by the end of next month', some effective affirmations might be:

1. 'I am a non-smoker and feel really healthy.'

2. 'I enjoy breathing in fresh, smoke-free air.'

Seeing is believing

Go confidently in the direction of your dreams. Live the life you've imagined!
Henry David Thoreau

We often describe our goals as dreams; this is because most of us imagine ourselves achieving them before we take action to make them happen. When you do this, your subconscious believes you have already achieved your goal and makes sure you act as if you have. So, to make your affirmation effective you need to visualise the image your words conjure up. Words create pictures, sounds and emotions.

Try this: To imprint your affirmation on your subconscious mind, read it out loud first, then close your eyes and imagine yourself experiencing your goal in detail, using as many of your senses as you can. How do you look, walk, and speak, now that you have reached your goal? How do you feel? Proud? Confident? Elated? Content? Feel the emotions you have attached to your goal. What can you hear? Hear your friends and family congratulating you; they might say: 'Well done', 'Congratulations', 'I knew you could do it'. Reading, picturing, feeling and hearing your affirmation will have a powerful effect on your subconscious mind. Your subconscious won't accept an affirmation overnight – repeat each affirmation as often as you can until your mind believes it is a reality – then you should soon find yourself adopting behaviours that support your new self-image.

Sample goal plan

Now we are going to put all of these steps together to see what a completed goal plan would look like:

Goal: To stop smoking by the end of next month.

Why I want to achieve it:
1. To feel healthier and live longer.

2. To look better.

3. To stop smelling of smoke.

Benefits:
1. I'll feel fitter and healthier.

2. I'll look healthier.

3. I'll save money.

Obstacles	Solutions
Smoking out of habit at the end of a meal.	Replace with a new habit like having a cup of tea, or doing the washing up.
Being tempted to smoke when I get withdrawal symptoms.	Find ways to deal with the withdrawal symptoms, such as deep breathing, going for a walk and inhaling lavender oil to relax. Tell myself my withdrawal symptoms will pass soon.

First steps	Date Completed
Register with a smoking cessation service.	6 April
Decide which route to take, e.g. whether to use nicotine replacement therapy or another treatment.	11 April

Daily success habits:

1. Remind myself of the benefits of stopping smoking.

2. Go for a walk every day to take my mind off smoking and feel fitter and healthier.

Weekly success habits:

1. Attend my weekly smoking cessation clinic for support.

2. Buy myself a small treat with the money I've saved.

Deadline: 30 June.

Affirmation 1: 'I am a non-smoker. I look and feel great.'

Affirmation 2: 'I say "no" to cigarettes.'

Blank goal plan (for your use)

Goal..

Why I want to achieve it:

1. ....

2. ....

3. ....

Benefits:

1. ....

2. ....

3. ....

Obstacles	Solutions

First steps	Date Completed

Daily success habits:

1. ....

2. ....

3. ....

Weekly success habits:

1. ....

2. ....

3. ....

Deadline: ....

Affirmation 1: ....

....

Affirmation 2: ....

....

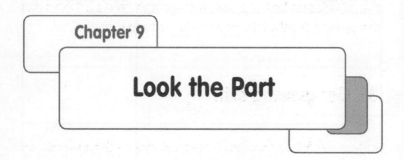

Chapter 9

Look the Part

As well as making sure that you feel great on the inside – both physically and mentally – it's also vital that you look good on the outside. Your outward appearance should reflect your new inner confidence and self-respect. Knowing that you are looking your best can help you to face the world with confidence and – like it or not – we are all judged on our appearance.

Confidence in how you look comes from making the most of what you have, not from trying to drastically alter your looks, or aiming to look like a carbon copy of someone else. Anyone can look good if they eat a nutritious diet, take regular exercise, look after their skin, hair and nails, and choose a hairstyle and clothes that suit them; you can also use cosmetics to accentuate your best features, camouflage any imperfections and generally enhance your appearance.

This chapter offers you simple but effective skin care, hair care and style tips to help you look polished, stylish and full of confidence.

Look your best

When you know that you are looking your best you can't help but feel more confident in any situation. Looking your best doesn't have to involve following complicated skin and hair care routines and using expensive products; to keep your skin and hair in peak condition, all you need to do is keep them cleansed and moisturised. Remember that to look their best your skin, hair and nails need a balanced diet that provides healthy fats, protein, vitamins and minerals.

37. Get glowing skin

Rather than following a complicated skin care routine that involves using lots of different products and takes a lot of time, focus on the four key steps:

1. Cleanse – to remove any dirt from your skin.

2. Exfoliate – to gently slough away dead skin cells to reveal the brighter 'newer' skin beneath.

3. Tone – to close the pores and leave your skin fresh and glowing.

4. Moisturise – to lock in moisture and form a protective barrier on your skin.

You can do these four steps using just one or two products if you are short of time or money.

There is a bewildering array of skin care products on the market. The secret is to choose products that suit your skin type and budget.

Identify your skin type

Most people have one of four basic skin types: dry, normal, oily or combination. Dry skin usually has a fine, matte texture and tends to be sensitive, and more prone to redness, flakiness, fine lines and wrinkles than other skin types. Normal skin has no dry or greasy areas and has an even tone. Oily skin looks greasy first thing in the morning and even an hour after cleansing. It is more prone to open pores, spots and blackheads than other skin types, but on the plus side it's also less susceptible to fine lines and wrinkles. Combination skin, as the name suggests, is a mixture of both oily and normal/dry skin; usually the forehead, nose and chin are greasy and the cheeks are normal or dry.

Buy products to suit your skin and budget

Once you've identified your skin type buy yourself a suitable cleanser and moisturiser. There are lots of products out there containing everything from antioxidants to retinol (a form of vitamin A) all claiming to do amazing things, but dermatologists say that cheaper brands such as Simple or pharmacy own brands are just as good as the more expensive ones; all cleansing lotions and moisturisers are basically a mixture of water and oil.

If you're on a very tight budget buy one product that can multitask. For example, you could use a light lotion or, if your skin is dry, a heavier cream that can be used as a facial cleanser, eye make-up remover, moisturiser, body lotion, hand cream and even as a hydrating face mask if you apply extra: leave it on while you're in the bath or shower and then rinse it off with tepid water.

Sun protection

UV radiation from the sun damages the elastin and collagen fibres in the skin, causing lasting damage and premature ageing. Most dermatologists agree that the best way to prevent wrinkles is to protect your skin from the sun. Wear a moisturiser or foundation with a minimum sun protection factor (SPF) of 15 every day. Always apply sun cream to your body prior to exposure and reapply frequently. Choose products with both UVA and UVB protection to protect your body from the ageing and burning effects of the sun. For the best protection experts recommend applying sun cream liberally and avoid rubbing it in too much. Avoid the sun's rays between 10am and 3pm as this is the time when they are at their strongest. Cover up, or stay in the shade, but remember the sun's rays reflect off water, sand and snow, so still wear protection.

> ### How to cleanse, tone and moisturise with one product
>
> Step 1: Massage in lotion or cream to cleanse.
> Step 2: Remove with a damp facecloth, or muslin cloth, to remove dirt and exfoliate.
> Step 3: Splash with cold water to tone.
> Step 4: Reapply cream or lotion to moisturise. If you have greasy skin, apply sparingly. If you have combination skin, only apply to the drier areas.

38. Have heavenly hair

Your hair is one of the first things people notice about you, so make sure yours is in great shape by having regular trims and taking good care of it.

Go for a style that suits your hair type and emphasises natural curls, waves or straight hair, so that you don't spend hours battling against nature with straighteners, perms or lots of styling products. Avoid getting stuck in a time warp; if you've had the same hair style for years, getting a new cut can give you a huge confidence boost. Find a hair stylist you feel listens to you. Take pictures to give an idea of the look you're after. Ask for advice on which cuts will suit your face shape, hair type and age. Top stylists recommend a trim every six weeks, to avoid split ends and to keep your hair looking its best.

As with skin care products, you don't need to go for expensive shampoos and conditioners; according to beauty experts all shampoos contain the same basic ingredients, regardless of how much they cost. Again, the key is to choose products that suit your hair type, i.e. dry, greasy, normal, coloured or to tackle problems like dandruff. It is also important to use a conditioner after every shampoo to smooth the hairs' cuticles and moisturise the hair. This helps to protect the hair from damage, and keep it soft and shiny.

Again, if you are on a tight budget go for multitasking products where possible; for example, baby shampoo has a multitude of uses: not only will it effectively cleanse your hair, but it also makes a great, gentle body wash, foam bath, face wash and even eye make-up remover, and lathered up makes a great shaving foam.

When you apply conditioner, concentrate on the mid-lengths and ends. Rinse well, finishing with cool water. For extra deep conditioning, cover your hair with a plastic cap or bag after applying conditioner and leave it on while you take your shower or bath. The plastic traps heat which opens the cuticles and allows the treatment to penetrate deeper.

If you're short of time, use a leave-in conditioner to avoid having to rinse your hair twice. Use cold water for the final rinse; it smooths the hair cuticles so they reflect light for super-shiny hair. If you run out of conditioner, use vinegar in the final rinse; simply add a tablespoon to a one-litre jug of lukewarm water; it works by restoring the hair's natural acid balance and removing dulling products from the hair. Ordinary malt vinegar will do, but white vinegar or apple cider vinegar work equally well.

End with a tiny amount of serum, to protect your hair from styling aids, prevent dryness and flyaway hair, and add shine.

Top styling tips

 Use a wide-tooth comb to gently tease out tangles.

 Allow your hair to air dry for a few minutes or rough dry it with the dryer.

 Hold the hairdryer at least 6 inches away from your hair, beginning on a high speed and temperature, and lowering the heat as your hair dries.

 Dry one section at a time, in the opposite direction to the way it usually falls, with a round brush to create movement and a smooth finish.

 Stop blow-drying when your hair is just dry to help avoid damage and breakage.

 Hair straighteners create a sleek, shiny look, but overusing them can cause damage and breakage. Only use them on dry hair; avoid going over the same area twice or straightening right to the ends as these are the most fragile sections of the hair.

39. Care for your hands and nails

Like your skin and hair, your hands are constantly on display, so to feel totally confident about your appearance you need to make sure they look well cared for.

1. **Protect your hands** – from hot water and household chemicals, by wearing rubber gloves when you do household chores. During the winter, wear gloves to shield your hands from the elements.

2. **Use a gentle moisturising soap or handwash** – that strips away fewer of your natural oils.

3. **Replace lost moisture** – with regular applications of hand cream; carry a tube around with you. Apply extra cream to the backs of your hands, where the skin is thinner, and in between your fingers, where the skin is prone to cracking and chapping.

4. **Use a moisturising hand scrub** – to remove dead, dry skin cells, cleanse and hydrate. Mix a little sugar, or salt with enough olive or rapeseed oil to make a thick paste; massage in for a minute or two, then rinse off to leave your hands looking and feeling soft and smooth.

Nail it

Bitten-down finger nails not only look awful, they also suggest that their owner is nervous and lacking in confidence. Try these tips to help you give up the habit.

1. Use a bitter-tasting nail-biting deterrent, such as Stop'n Grow, or wear a pretty nail varnish; you'll find it harder to bite lacquered nails.

2. Keep your nails trimmed short, so that you have less nail to chew.

3. Have a nail file or clippers to hand at all times to deal with snags and splits straight away, as these often give an 'excuse' for nail-biting.

4. Look after your nails; then you will feel less inclined to bite them. Massage hand cream or olive oil into your nails and cuticles every night before bed, to keep them in good condition.

40. Style yourself confident

What you wear both reflects how you feel about yourself and your life, and affects how others perceive you. Someone who believes they are unattractive might express this by wearing loose, frumpy clothing; a person lacking confidence might dress head to toe in black, grey or neutral colours to avoid drawing attention to themselves. You can change your self-concept and how other people see you simply by changing the way you dress. To feel confident you need to feel comfortable and happy with what you are wearing, as well as create the right impression; below are the key elements you should take into account if you want to style yourself confident.

1. **Your age** – whether you are male or female, avoid dressing too young or too old for your age. This doesn't mean you can't wear fashionable clothes just because you are a certain age, but it does mean recognising that your body shape and role in life change as you grow older, and this should be reflected in the clothes you choose.

2. **Your shape** – choose clothes that fit well and flatter your shape. Avoid wearing baggy clothes to hide a big chest, tummy

or wide hips; rather than disguising the problem area they can make you look large all over. Fitted clothes are far more flattering, whatever your size or shape. A tailored jacket, dress or blouse that goes in at the waist can give the illusion of an hour-glass shape even if you don't have one. For men, pinstripe suits and vertically striped dress shirts can make you look taller and slimmer; if you have a large rear avoid wearing double vented jackets – stick to single or non-vented styles that are long enough to cover your bottom. If you have a large tummy, avoid shirts or tee shirts with 'busy' prints, as these will draw attention to your upper body; opt for plain colours or subtle patterns instead.

3. **Your personality and personal taste** – the style of clothes you choose should say something about your sense of self and your personal taste. For example, your style might be, classic, trendy, sporty, casual, feminine, romantic, masculine or bold.

4. **The occasion** – as well as portraying your personality, to feel confident and project the right image your clothes need to suit the occasion, but you can still reveal your personality and sense of style for example, if your style is sporty and casual you might feel more comfortable – and confident – in a smart trouser suit with flat shoes for a job interview, whereas if you are prefer a more feminine style you could wear a skirt suit, or a smart dress and jacket with heels. A man who prefers a classic style might opt for a traditional suit, whereas someone who likes to be trendy might choose the latest fashion from their favourite designer. The trick is to adapt your personal taste to suit the occasion.

5. **Which colours and shades suit you** – One of the secrets to looking and feeling your best is to wear colours that complement your skin tone, hair colour and body shape. A

splash of colour can make you look younger and boost your confidence. To find out which colours suit you best try this exercise: choose clothes from your wardrobe in the colours you wear most often and sort them into piles according to colour. Stand in front of a full-length mirror in daylight. Taking one colour at a time hold each garment next to your face and note the effects; the right colours and shades will enliven your skin, brighten your eyes and complement your hair colour, while the wrong ones will leave your complexion looking washed out, your eyes dull and your hair colour flat. Bear in mind that whilst one shade of a particular colour, say navy blue, may not flatter you at all, another shade, say turquoise blue, might.

Another point to consider when choosing which colours to wear is the effect different colours can have on how you feel and act; for example blue and green are considered calming, whilst yellow can lift your mood and red can make you feel confident and energetic. Most people can wear most colours; it's just a case of choosing the best shade for your colouring. Remember, too, that darker shades are usually more figure-flattering than lighter hues.

When you know that what you are wearing suits both your style and the situation and also enhances your best features, you can't help but feel at ease, authentic and confident.

Chapter 10

Try Confidence-Boosting DIY Complementary Therapies

Complementary therapies – also known as complementary or alternative medicine, or natural or holistic therapies – aim to identify and rectify the causes of illness and treat the whole person, whereas conventional Western medicine only treats the symptoms of ill-health, not the individual. More and more people, concerned about side-effects from prescribed drugs, are turning to complementary therapies to reduce stress and to improve their general physical and mental wellbeing, or to help them manage chronic health conditions.

The words 'health' and 'healing' are derived from the Old English word 'hale', which means wholeness. Complementary therapies are based on this idea that health is about wholeness and that total wellbeing is achieved when the self as a whole – mind, body and spirit – are in a state of balance known as homeostasis. They view illness as a sign that this harmony has been disrupted, and attempt to restore good health by stimulating the body's natural self-healing and self-regulating abilities.

Homeostasis can be achieved by following the type of lifestyle recommended in this book, i.e. a wholesome diet with plenty of fresh air, exercise, rest, relaxation and sleep, combined with stress management and a positive mental attitude. Complementary therapies such as aromatherapy, massage and reflexology can help you to achieve homeostasis by relaxing the muscles, easing mental stress, promoting relaxation and improving sleep.

Whether complementary therapies work or not remains under debate. Some argue that any benefits from such therapies are down to the placebo effect, which is where a treatment improves symptoms simply because the person using it believes it will, rather than because it has any real therapeutic effect.

However, there is growing evidence that the mind and body are inextricably linked, and that mental stresses and strains can affect physical health, while physical health problems can affect mental health. For example, stress can trigger conditions like IBS, migraine, eczema and even heart disease, while people suffering from diseases like arthritis, heart disease, or cancer often suffer from depression and low self-esteem or confidence. Also, it could be argued that, unlike relatively new drug treatments, complementary therapies have stood the test of time, having been used to treat ailments and promote wellbeing for thousands of years.

This chapter gives you an overview of some of the complementary therapies that could boost your confidence by enhancing your overall health and wellbeing, and includes techniques and treatments you can try for yourself, including the Alexander Technique, aromatherapy, massage, emotional freedom techniques (EFT), Bach Flower Remedies, homeopathy and herbal supplements.

41. Perfect your posture with the Alexander Technique

We have already discussed how you can instantly boost your self-confidence by adopting a 'power posture' in Action 22; now we are going to look at how the Alexander Technique can also help you to improve the way you hold and move your body as you go about your daily life. Also, as with the 'power pose', when you hold yourself well people will perceive you as a confident person.

The technique teaches you to pay attention to your posture, movement and thinking, as well as any tension in your body, and how to overcome unhelpful habits. Because the technique encourages you to focus on how your body is feeling *now* it also helps you to live in the present, which benefits you psychologically. Teachers of the Alexander Technique claim that the key benefits include feeling more confident and empowered, as well as enjoying better concentration and feeling more relaxed.

The technique was developed in the 1890s by Australian actor Frederick Matthias Alexander, when he noticed he was tensing his muscles and adopting an unnatural posture in response to physical and emotional stress before a show, and that this was having a negative effect on his performance.

Poor posture can also lead to neck, shoulder and back pain and headaches, which could also sap your confidence; the Alexander Technique aims to improve posture and enable the body to function with the minimum amount of strain on the joints and muscles, helping to relieve muscular tension and pain. It does this by restoring the correct positioning of the head, neck and back, the core of the body.

To ensure that you adopt the correct posture, it's best to learn the Alexander Technique from a qualified teacher. A teacher will assess your posture and movement, and demonstrate how you can rectify any bad habits so that you can move more freely and naturally. Once you have become proficient you will be able to practise at home. Your ultimate aim will be to hold your body in the correct stance all the time. However, in the meantime, here are three techniques you can try to help you regain your natural poise, prevent and ease muscular tension, and crank up your self-confidence.

Stand up straight

1. Stand with your hands by your sides and your feet hip-width apart, with your weight distributed equally between both feet.

2. Ensure your knees feel relaxed, not 'locked' backwards.

3. Imagine the crown (upper back) of your head being pulled upwards, letting your chin drop and your forehead roll slightly forwards. Allow your shoulders to relax.

4. Focus your body weight to fall mainly on your heels and ensure your upper body is facing straight ahead.

Walk tall

1. Adopt the standing pose outlined above.

2. As you walk, concentrate on your weight shifting from one foot to the other, making each movement as effortless as you can. Again, your heels should support most of your weight.

3. Hold your upper body upright, not leaning forwards.

4. Lead each step with a foot, not your chin or torso.

Let go of muscular tension

1. Identify which muscles are tense.

2. One by one, mentally tell each muscle to 'let go', imagining the tension draining away.

42. Use aroma power

Aromatherapy is based on the idea that inhaling the scents released from essential oils affects the hypothalamus – the part of the brain that controls the glands and hormones – triggering the release of neurotransmitters and endorphins, and thus altering mood. As well as affecting the emotions, many oils also possess healing or anti-inflammatory, pain-relieving properties. When used in massage, baths and compresses, oils are also absorbed through the skin into the bloodstream and transported to muscles, organs and glands, which are believed to benefit from their therapeutic effects.

There is a growing body of evidence to support these claims; a study in 2005 at the Medical University of Vienna, Austria, reported that participants who were exposed to floral scents used three times more positive words in written tests than those who weren't. In 2009, Japanese researchers found that linalool, a component of lavender, lemon, orange and basil essential oils, lowers levels of the stress hormone cortisol in the blood stream. The mental health charity Mind recognises the relaxing and stress-relieving effects of aromatherapy.

How to use aromatherapy oils:

Massage:
A two per cent dilution is usually used for massage: this equates to two drops of essential oil for each teaspoon of carrier oil. Stronger oils may need to be diluted more; this is mentioned where necessary in the following information. Sweet almond and grapeseed oils are popular carrier oils, but you could also use good quality olive, sunflower, or sesame oil from your kitchen. See Action 43 for more information on massage.

Safety advice:
Never apply aromatherapy oils to broken skin. Buy the best quality essential oils you can afford; like most things, you get what you pay for; cheaper oils may not be as pure as more expensive ones and are

more likely to be mixed with solvents or synthetic oils. If you have sensitive skin it is a good idea to do a patch test before using an essential oil you haven't used before; apply a few drops of diluted oil to the inside of a wrist or elbow, or behind an earlobe. If there is no reaction within 24 hours it should be safe to go ahead and use the oil. Even diluted oils should be kept away from the eyes and out of reach of children.

Aromatic bath:
Fill the bath with comfortably hot water. Just before you get in, add six drops of your chosen essential oil (unless otherwise stated). Agitate the water with your hand to disperse the oil, which will then form a thin film on the water. The warmth of the water both aids absorption through the skin and releases the aromatic vapours, which are then inhaled.

Steam inhalation:
This method is very effective for clearing your head or your nasal passages, or for relieving a headache. Add three to four drops of your chosen oil to a bowl of very hot, but not boiling, water. Lean over the bowl and carefully drape a large towel around your head and the bowl. Inhale the vapours for a minute or two.
Caution: Supervise children while using this method, to ensure they don't scald themselves.

Hot compress:
A hot compress is a great way of easing tense, aching muscles especially in the neck, shoulders and back, and also works well for headaches. The warmth from the compress releases the aromatic vapours and assists absorption through the pores. Soak a facecloth or handkerchief in a basin of hot water to which you have added four or five drops of your chosen oil. Wring out the excess moisture and apply to the painful area.

Tip: For a quick and easy way to enjoy your favourite essential oil, add about 20 drops to a bottle of your favourite shower gel or bath foam. Shake well before each use.

The best oils for boosting self-confidence are those with stimulating, uplifting, calming or relaxing properties. Below is a selection of oils with one or more of these actions, with references to some of their other general uses:

Bergamot
Bergamot's citrus aroma is uplifting, and it also has relaxing and calming effects.
Caution: Use in one per cent dilution, as in higher strengths it can make your skin more sensitive to sunlight and more likely to burn.

Clary sage
Clary sage has a nutty aroma and is a powerful muscle relaxant and de-stressor, encouraging restful sleep.

Geranium
This floral-scented oil balances the emotions and uplifts; it can have a stimulating effect on the mind, so it is best to avoid using it within three hours or so of bedtime.

Peppermint
Cooling peppermint stimulates and energises the mind, as well as clearing the head; it can also ease the pain of headaches and migraines, and soothe an upset stomach; use a one per cent dilution in a carrier oil and massage gently into the stomach and abdomen. Drinking peppermint tea as well will augment the effects. Avoid using peppermint within three hours of bedtime as it can promote wakefulness.

Rosemary

This pungent oil has a stimulant effect on the mind, boosting concentration and memory, and also eases muscular pain and symptoms of the common cold.

Caution: If you suffer from epileptic fits avoid using rosemary oil.

Vetiver

Known as 'the oil of tranquility' in India, vetiver calms and relaxes, helping to ease stress and anxiety and to induce sound sleep.

43. Enjoy a mood-lifting massage

Massage is probably the oldest technique used for promoting and maintaining general wellbeing, and no doubt developed from our natural instinct to rub a painful area, or our innate need to show affection through touch. There's evidence that ancient civilisations such as the Egyptians, Romans and Greeks used massage for its pain-relieving and relaxing properties. The ancient Greek doctor Hippocrates – often referred to as the 'father of medicine' – suggested that he used massage on his patients when he wrote: 'The physician must be qualified in many things, but most assuredly in rubbing.'

Massage triggers the release of serotonin and endorphins, which not only help to relax the mind and ease pain, but also boost your mood and therefore your confidence. Massage also relieves the stress-related muscular tension that can build up in the neck and shoulders, loosens and stretches the muscles and boosts the circulation. Ask your partner or a friend to give you a massage and then offer to reciprocate; warm your chosen massage oil between your palms before applying to the neck, shoulders and back, using one or more of these basic massage techniques:

Stroking/effleurage – aids circulation and relaxes tense muscles; use gentle to firm pressure as you move both hands over the skin in rhythmic fanning or circular movements.

 Kneading/petrissage – stretches and relaxes the muscles; use your thumbs and fingers to squeeze then release the flesh, as if you are kneading dough.

Friction – is used on the back and shoulders to release tension from the muscles; use your thumbs to apply even pressure in small, circular movements.

Hacking – use the sides of your outstretched hands alternately to deliver short, sharp taps all over the body.

44. Tap into emotional freedom techniques (EFT)

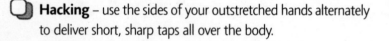

The emotional freedom techniques (EFT), like acupressure and acupuncture, are energy therapies based on meridian theory; this is the belief that life energy, or qi, flows along 22 channels in the body known as meridians. An even passage of qi throughout the body is viewed as vital for good health. Disruption of the flow of qi in a meridian can lead to illness at any point within it. The passage of qi can be affected by various psychological and lifestyle factors, including stress, emotional distress, diet and environment. Because of the similarities between EFT and acupressure, they are often known as 'psychological acupressure'.

According to EFT, many of us hold on to negative emotions, which are then stored in the meridians where they stop the flow of energy and encourage more negative thoughts. The techniques are derived from the Chinese system of chi kung, which involves tapping on particular points to rebalance the energy flow throughout the body.

In EFT you repeat a statement out loud that describes your negative emotions in a way that makes you feel more positive and promotes self-acceptance, while tapping specific points on your meridians. It is claimed that this sends a pulse of energy through the meridians, which releases your negative emotions.

A similar technique, known as thought field therapy (TFT), has been adapted and used by well-known hypnotherapist Paul McKenna to help people overcome insomnia, stress and worry. Celebrity fans of EFT include Madonna, Lily Allen and Michael Ball. To use the techniques to boost your confidence try this:

1. Focus on a negative emotion that is affecting your confidence. For example: 'I am frightened to go for what I want in case I fail.' Then rate how strongly you feel the emotion out of 10, with 0 being the lowest score and 10 being the highest. Next, to help you feel more positive about yourself, and to practise self-acceptance, reframe this statement with the words 'Even though... I deeply love and accept myself', so that the statement becomes: 'Even though I am frightened to go for what I want in case I fail, I deeply love and accept myself'.

2. Using the tips of your index and middle fingers, tap five times on the 'side of eye' meridian points, situated on the outer bony part of the eye sockets, where the eyebrows end. Stimulating this point is said to promote calm. As you tap, repeat your statement, so that you focus on the negative beliefs or thoughts you have about yourself.

3. Using your right index and middle fingers, tap five times on the left 'underarm' meridian point, situated under your armpit,

in line with your nipple. Repeat on your right side using your left index and middle fingers. Stimulating these points is said to relieve worry, aid concentration and speed up thought processes. As you tap, repeat your statement to help you focus on the negative thoughts or beliefs you want to let go of.

4. At the end of the tapping sequence, rate the strength of your emotion again. You should notice that your rating has dropped. Repeat the sequence using the same statement until your rating is a low as you can get it at that point.

5. Finally, repeat the sequence again but with a new, more positive statement that includes a description of how you want to feel. For example: 'Even though I still feel a little afraid, I accept that fear is normal and I choose to go for what I want.'

For more information and an EFT tapping points diagram, go to www.theenergytherapycentre.co.uk/tapping-points.htm.

45. Try flower power

Flower essences have been used for their healing properties for thousands of years. However, it was Dr Edward Bach, a Harley Street doctor, bacteriologist and homeopath, who developed their use in the twentieth century. He was one of the first modern medical practitioners to treat the causes of disease rather than just the symptoms.

Bach believed that negative emotions could cause illness and that the mind, body and spirit had to be in total harmony for physical and mental wellbeing. He also thought that flowers had healing properties which could be used to relieve emotional problems and thus restore good health. He identified 38 basic negative states of mind and created a plant or flower-based remedy for each. The remedies are designed to promote wellbeing by combating negative emotions, such as fear, despair and uncertainty, and encouraging a positive frame of mind. Whilst research suggests that a healthy mind does help to ensure a healthy body, there is only anecdotal evidence that Bach Flower Remedies are effective.

The remedies are made by soaking flower heads in spring water in direct sunlight, or by boiling twigs from trees, bushes or plants. Brandy is added to the infusion to preserve the mixture and form a tincture. The remedies can be taken mixed with water, or you can use them neat dropped onto your tongue or rubbed into your lips, temples, wrists or behind your ears. They're widely available in pharmacies in handy-sized 10 ml and 20 ml phials. Below is a list of Bach Remedies that you may find helpful when your self-confidence needs a boost.

- **Bach Rescue Remedy** – this combination of rock rose, impatiens, clematis, star of Bethlehem and cherry plum is designed to steady the emotions and to restore inner calm, control and focus at times of acute stress, such as before an exam or job interview. It is also available as a spray and a cream (which also contains crab apple), pastilles and chewing gum.

- **Crab apple** – good for people who have a poor self-image; especially if they are ashamed or embarrassed by their physical appearance. Helps to overcome self-loathing and low self-esteem.

- **Larch** – good for boosting confidence before an exam, interview or driving test, etc. Helps people to have more confidence in their abilities, overcome their fear of failure and reach their full potential.

📋 **Mimulus** – helps to dispel fears and worries that hold us back and stop us doing the things we would like to do, and encourages a positive frame of mind.

📋 **Cerato** – helps those who lack confidence in their own judgement, especially when making decisions.

For further information on how to select a suitable flower remedy, and an online questionnaire that enables you to select a personalised blend, visit www.bachfloweressences.co.uk.

46. Get help from homeopathy

Homeopathy was founded by the eighteenth-century German physician Dr Samuel Hahnemann, who was so unhappy with conventional medicine he began looking for a safer, gentler approach to healing.

Homeopathy means 'same suffering' and is based on the idea that 'like cures like'; substances that in large amounts can cause symptoms in a well person can, in small amounts, treat the same symptoms in a person who is ill. For example, coffee contains caffeine, which in excess can over-stimulate the mind and cause nervousness and insomnia, so the remedy coffea is often prescribed for these very symptoms.

According to homeopaths, symptoms such as inflammation and fever are signs that the body is trying to heal itself. They believe that homeopathic remedies encourage this self-healing process and work rather like a vaccination, because their effects mimic those of the illness they are designed to treat. This approach is completely the opposite to conventional medicines which aim to suppress symptoms.

Homeopathic remedies are made from plant, animal, mineral and metal sources. These substances are mixed with a solution of alcohol and water, and left to stand for several days or even weeks. The mixture is then strained through a filter, or squeezed through a press to produce a liquid known as the 'mother tincture'. One drop of the mother tincture is then diluted with pure alcohol and distilled water and succussed, i.e. shaken vigorously, or banged on a hard surface, many times over to increase its potency. Once the mixture is at the right dilution and potency a few drops are added to base tablets.

Paradoxically, homeopaths claim that the more diluted a remedy is, the greater its healing properties and the fewer its potential side-effects. They say this is due to the 'memory of water', i.e. the belief that even though the molecules from a substance are highly diluted, they leave behind an electromagnetic 'footprint' – like a recording on an audiotape – which has the same effect on the body as the original substance.

There are two main types of remedies; whole-person based and symptom based. It's probably best to consult a qualified homeopath who will prescribe a remedy aimed at you as a whole person, based on your personality, as well as your symptoms. However, if you prefer, you can buy homeopathic remedies at many high street pharmacies and health shops.

These ideas are controversial and many GPs remain sceptical; a report in 2009 by the Science and Technology Committee of the UK Parliament concluded that while some homeopathic remedies appeared to make patients feel better, it was likely this was due to the placebo effect. However, the British Homeopathic Society argues that there is a growing body of evidence to show homeopathy has a beneficial effect on 77 different health problems including depression, anxiety and insomnia.

Below are details of two homeopathic remedies that are claimed to help treat a lack of self-confidence:

Anacardium Orientale
Made from: Marking nuts, which grow in India, Malaysia and Indonesia.
Emotional symptoms: Low self-confidence; inferiority complex.
Symptoms improved by: Exposure to sunshine.
Symptoms made worse by: Stress; fear.

Lycopodium
Made from: Plant commonly known as club moss or stag's horn moss, which is found growing on moorland and in woodland.
Emotional symptoms: Lack of self-confidence; fear of failing.
Symptoms improved by: Outdoor exercise.
Symptoms made worse by: Inactivity.

Not a quick fix

Practitioners warn that homeopathy isn't a quick fix; the remedies may take a while to work. Homeopathic remedies are generally considered safe and don't have any known side effects, although sometimes a temporary worsening of symptoms known as 'aggravation' may take place. This is seen as a good sign, as it suggests that the remedy is stimulating the healing process. If this happens, stop taking the remedy and wait for your symptoms to improve. If there is steady improvement, don't restart the remedy. If the improvement stops, start taking the remedy again. You may see an improvement within hours, or it could take several weeks or even months, depending on whether your condition is acute or chronic.

47. Try confidence-boosting herbal supplements

If you have followed some of the suggestions in this book, but still feel that you need a little extra help in boosting your confidence, you could consider trying a herbal supplement. The most beneficial herbal supplements for increasing confidence are those that boost mood and concentration, relieve stress, and promote calm and sound sleep.

Do supplements work?

Often there is only anecdotal evidence that a supplement works. While you need to be cautious about unsupported claims, bear in mind that sometimes the lack of evidence is simply down to the fact that the research hasn't been done. Even though the turnover in the herbal medicine sector is quite high, many manufacturers cannot meet the high costs of clinical trials, so a lack of evidence to back up the use of a supplement doesn't necessarily mean it doesn't work, or isn't safe, but it is important to exercise caution and make sure you only buy products from reputable companies.

Another issue is that some herbal remedies have several active ingredients and this can make it difficult to identify which produce the beneficial effects. Also, the quality of herbal medicines can vary due to differences in plant species, the type of soil they are grown in, extraction methods and storage, etc. These variations can sometimes make it hard to draw firm conclusions about particular herbs.

It is reassuring to know that the Medicines and Healthcare products Regulatory Agency (MHRA) has recently tightened up the regulation of herbal medicines and supplements to help ensure their effectiveness, safety and quality (see page 126).

Are herbal supplements safe to use?

It is important to remember that just because something is termed 'natural' it is not necessarily harmless. Herbs contain chemicals that have an effect on the body, just as drugs do, and herbal medicines are subject to legislation to help ensure the safety of the people who use them. If you are taking prescribed medications, speak to your GP before taking a herbal supplement to make sure it won't affect their potency or effectiveness, or cause harmful side effects.

Find out more about herbal supplements

MHRA provides a list of herbal products currently registered under the Traditional Herbal Medicines Registration Scheme, along with information sheets on their safe use. You can also report any adverse reactions herbal remedies or supplements may have caused to the agency. The agency's contact details can be found in the Directory at the end of this book.

Regulation of herbal medicines

According to the MHRA, a herbal medicine is any medicinal product that contains one or more herbal substances as active ingredients, one or more herbal preparations, or a combination of the two. Since April 2011, all herbal medicines have had to be registered under the Traditional Herbal Medicines Registration Scheme, or hold a product licence. Registered herbal medicines have to meet specific safety and quality standards and carry agreed indications for when and how they should be used. Licensed herbal medicines have to meet certain standards of safety, quality and effectiveness. For more information go to: www.mhra.gov.uk/howweregulate/medicines/herbalmedicinesregulation/registeredtraditionalherbalmedicines/index.htm.

Here is an overview of four herbal supplements that have properties that could help to improve your confidence: 5-HTP, passion flower, rhodiola rosea and valerian. They are available in various forms, including capsules, tablets and tinctures. Related products are listed below and further details are given in the Useful Products section at the end of the book.

5-Hydroxytryptophan (5-HTP)

What it is: 5-HTP is a supplement usually made from the seeds of the griffonia plant, which comes from West Africa.

Confidence-boosting effects: It boosts mood, relieves anxiety and panic attacks, and promotes sound sleep.

How it works: The body uses 5-HTP to produce the 'happy hormone' serotonin, a lack of which is linked with low mood, anxiety and poor sleep. Serotonin is also converted into the 'sleep hormone' melatonin.

Evidence it works: Several small studies suggest that 5-HTP may be as effective as some antidepressant drugs for the relief of mild to moderate depression; one study involving 63 people compared the effects of 5-HTP to fluvoxamine (Luvox), an SSRI (selective serotonin reuptake inhibitor), which is a type of antidepressant that increases the level of serotonin in the blood. Those who were given 5-HTP did just as well as those who received Luvox and suffered fewer side effects. In another study, people who took 5-HTP fell asleep more easily and slept more soundly than those who took a placebo.

Safety: 5-HTP should not be taken with SSRI antidepressants such as Prozac, with weight-control drugs, triptans (medication used to treat migraines) or the painkiller tramadol. Nor should it be taken

if you are pregnant. Some people may experience a temporary worsening of anxiety symptoms before noticing an improvement.
Available as: Tablets, such as Healthspan 5-HTP 100 mg, Serotone 5-HTP and Solgar 5 Hydroxytryptophan.

Passion flower
What it is: Passion flower is a climbing shrub with purple and white flowers that is native to South America and popular with gardeners in the UK. Both the flowers and leaves can be used. It is also known as passiflora.
Confidence-boosting effects: Passion flower combats stress and helps to calm the nerves. It is also a traditional South African remedy for insomnia, especially for people who have trouble staying asleep.
How it works: Its active ingredients are alkaloids, which have mildly sedative effects, possibly by enhancing the effects of the calming brain chemical gamma-aminobutyric acid (GABA).
Evidence it works: A small double-blind RCT in 2001 found it to be as effective as the tranquiliser oxazepam in the treatment of generalised anxiety, but with fewer side effects.
Safety: Passion flower may very occasionally cause dizziness, confusion, heart problems and inflammation of blood vessels. Very rarely, there may be toxicity, even with normal doses. Do not take passion flower if you are pregnant or breastfeeding.
Available as: Tablets (e.g. RelaxHerb), a liquid extract (Passiflora and Valerian Plus) and a tincture (e.g. from G Baldwin & Co and Napiers).

Rhodiola rosea
What it is: Rhodiola rosea is an extract from the rhizome or root of the rhodiola plant, which grows in Scandinavia, Canada, Siberia and northern China. It is also known as golden root.
Confidence-boosting effects: It relieves symptoms of stress, such as mild anxiety, and boosts concentration.

How it works: The active ingredients are rosavins, which improve the body's ability to cope with physical, mental and environmental stress by acting on the hypothalamus. They may also help the transportation of mood-boosting tryptophan and 5-HTP to the brain.

Evidence it works: Various animal, laboratory and human studies have shown that rhodiola rosea can help to raise stress tolerance. A pilot six-week study, published in *The Journal of Alternative and Complementary Medicine* in 2008, suggested that a daily 340 mg dose of rhodiola rosea extract significantly reduced anxiety levels in ten participants who had been diagnosed with general anxiety.

Safety: Do not take rhodiola rosea if you are pregnant or suffer from kidney or liver problems.

Available as: Tablets (e.g. Vitano), capsules and an alcohol-free extract (e.g. from G Baldwin & Co).

Valerian

What it is: Valerian is a plant with pink and white flowers that is sometimes known as 'nature's valium'. The root is the part used in herbal medicine.

Confidence-boosting effects: It is thought to help relieve stress, worry and insomnia as well as boost mood.

How it works: Valerian seems to encourage the release of the neurotransmitter gamma-aminobutyric acid (GABA). It may also counteract the stimulant effects of caffeine.

Evidence it works: Valerian is a traditional herbal remedy for anxiety and is approved by the German E Commission (a German committee that reviews the quality, safety and effectiveness of herbal medicines) for use as a mild sedative. Some studies have found that valerian may relieve anxiety and others have not. In 2006, a systematic review of the evidence regarding how effective valerian is in the treatment of anxiety concluded that more, bigger RCTs were needed.

Safety: *Valeriana officinalis* is thought to be safe, but some other species of valerian may cause liver problems. Occasional side effects include drowsiness, mild headaches and nausea. Very rarely, there may be nervousness and excitability. Pregnant or breastfeeding women shouldn't take valerian, as there is a lack of information regarding safety. If you are taking any medications, speak to your GP or pharmacist first before using valerian as it can cause delirium when taken alongside loperamide, a drug used to treat diarrhoea, and fluoxetine, an SSRI antidepressant.

Available as: Tablets (e.g. Stressless and Kalms), a liquid extract (e.g. Passiflora and Valerian Plus) and a tincture (e.g. Dormeasan).

Check the benefits

Supplements can take up to three months to have a noticeable effect. If you don't feel calmer and more confident by then, consider not taking them. If you notice any adverse effects stop taking them immediately.

Chapter 11

Be Confident in Real-Life Situations

This chapter suggests how you can apply the techniques and ideas from this book to real-life situations that often challenge even the most confident person: public speaking, attending a job interview and going on a date. For each situation you will find a handy checklist to remind you of the appropriate tools you could use to help you stay calm and confident.

48. Speak in public confidently

Before your speech

1. **Know your subject** – make sure you know as much as possible about the topic you are going to talk about, so you are confident about your message. Identify the purpose of your speech and the key points. If you are worried about forgetting these, jot down brief reminders on postcards to use as prompts.

2. **Visualise yourself delivering your speech confidently** – imagine what you'll see, feel and hear. For example, your audience smiling and nodding because they are enjoying your

speech, you looking and feeling calm and relaxed. Hear the audience applauding at the end of your speech.

3. **Think positive thoughts** – about yourself and your audience. For example: 'I'm knowledgeable about my topic. I can give a good speech'; 'I can give my audience the information they want'; 'My audience will enjoy my talk'.

During your speech
1. **Adopt a power pose** – sit or stand tall, looking straight ahead at your audience. Take a deep breath and imagine you are inflating and taking up more space. Keep your shoulders relaxed and arms, legs, knees and feet apart. Use open gestures, keeping your hands apart (for more details see Action 22, Adopt confident body language).

2. **Use your confident 'chocolate' voice** – imagine you are eating chocolate or another food you like the taste of, breathe in, expanding your tummy, then say 'mmm' as you breathe out (see Action 23 for more details). Focus on speaking slowly; most people speak too quickly when they are nervous.

3. **Take a few deep breaths in and out** – before you start talking and whenever you feel nervous.

49. Perform well at a job interview

Before the interview
1. **Research the company** – find out as much as you can about your prospective employer.

2. **Practise your interview technique** – ask a partner or friend

to 'interview' you by asking you some likely questions, such as: 'Why do you want this job' and 'What do you consider to be your weaknesses?' Think of questions you could ask about the job and the company. Identify your relevant experience and strengths, and how you will demonstrate these during the interview.

3. **Choose a smart outfit to wear** – for most job interviews this is usually a smart suit if you are a man, or a skirt or trouser suit, or a plain dress and jacket if you are a woman. Make sure you look well-groomed and business-like, don't overdo make-up or jewellery.

4. **Visualise the interview going well** – imagine answering the interview panel's questions calmly and knowledgeably and asking relevant questions.

At the interview

1. **Take a few deep breaths in and out and think positively** – for example: 'I can do well in this interview'; 'I am capable of doing this job.'

2. **Use confident, open body language** – sit up straight and make eye contact when a member of the interview panel is speaking to you. Avoid speaking too quickly or fidgeting.

3. **Finally** – relax, be yourself and enjoy your interview!

50. Feel at ease on a date

Before your date

1. **Adopt a positive but realistic attitude** – your date must be interested in you to have asked you out, but don't expect to fall madly in love the first time you go out. Tell yourself if it goes

well it may lead to a long-term relationship and if it doesn't go so well you will hopefully still have had a nice time and learned a little more about what sort of partner you would like to meet.

2. **Visualise your date going well** – picture yourself radiating confidence and talking with ease on your date. Affirm to yourself: 'I radiate confidence and feel relaxed on my date.'

3. **Make sure you look your best** – choose an outfit you look good in and feel comfortable wearing. Pamper your skin, hair and nails, and perfect your hairstyle and make-up (if you wear it) before you go out so that you can forget about your appearance once you are on your date.

4. **If it's a first date, tell someone where you are going** – and meet in a public place to keep yourself safe.

During the date

1. **If you feel nervous take a few deep breaths** – take a moment to identify any tension in your body; imagine it melting away, then relax.

2. **Use open body language** – so that you look relaxed, confident and approachable.

3. **Smile** – this will help you to relax and will put your date at ease as well.

4. **Be yourself** – don't pretend to be someone you're not just to impress your date; if they are right for you they will like you just the way you are.

To conclude

This book has offered you lots of advice and ideas to help you boost your confidence, so hopefully you are feeling inspired and ready to make some changes to your lifestyle and the way you think about yourself; the following sections aim to help you do this. There are recipes to help you put the dietary advice into practice, as well as details of useful products, including the herbal supplements mentioned in Action 47, that you may want to try. There is also a list of books you may find helpful if you want to learn more about some of the topics covered in this book.

You'll also find the contact details, including the web addresses, of organisations that you may want to consult for further information and support.

Recipes

This section features recipes based on the dietary recommendations outlined in this book. All of the dishes are not only nutritious, but also delicious and quick and easy to prepare!

Turkey ragu with wholewheat pasta (serves 1)

In this recipe the turkey provides protein, which helps to keep you full, and tryptophan, from which the body makes the 'happy hormone' serotonin and 'sleep hormone' melatonin. The tomatoes, garlic, bay leaves and basil provide vitamins, minerals and antioxidants. The olive or rapeseed oil provides monounsaturated fats to lower cholesterol levels.

Ingredients

1 tbsp olive or rapeseed oil
110 g turkey breast, finely chopped
½ leek, roughly chopped
1 garlic clove, peeled and crushed
2 tbsp tomato puree
400 g can of chopped tomatoes
2 tbsp white wine vinegar
3 bay leaves
80 g wholewheat pasta of your choice
Handful of fresh basil leaves, torn

Method
Heat the oil in a frying pan over a high heat. Add the chopped turkey and fry for 2-3 minutes or until golden brown. Add the leek and garlic to the pan and cook for a further 2-3 minutes until pale golden. Add the tomato puree, tinned tomatoes, white wine vinegar, and bay leaves. Stir well, then simmer over a low heat for up to an hour, or until sauce is thickened. When the sauce is almost ready cook the wholewheat pasta according to the instructions on the packet. Place the pasta on the serving plate and then top with turkey ragu sauce. Finally tear the basil leaves and sprinkle over the top.

Peppered mackerel and leek spaghetti (serves 4)

In this recipe the mackerel is rich in omega-3 oil for brain and heart health. Both the mackerel and the wholewheat pasta boost B vitamin and serotonin levels and balance the blood sugar. The leek provides vitamins A, B6 and K and a range of minerals. The basil and chilli provide disease-busting phytochemicals (plant chemicals).

Ingredients
320 g wholewheat spaghetti
2 garlic cloves
1 red chilli
4 peppered mackerel fillets
4 tbsp extra virgin olive or rapeseed oil
1 medium-sized leek, sliced
Handful fresh basil leaves, torn

Method
Cook the wholewheat spaghetti according to the instructions on the packet. Skin and crush the garlic and peel and finely chop the chilli. Cut the mackerel into 2.5-cm pieces. Heat the oil in a large frying pan or wok and fry the sliced leek until softened. Add the garlic and

chilli and fry gently for a further minute. Add the mackerel pieces and cook gently for 2 minutes or until heated through. Add the drained pasta to the mackerel and leek mixture. Toss the ingredients together over a low heat, ensuring that the pasta is hot and well coated in the oil. Place on the serving plates and garnish with torn basil leaves.

Spicy chicken noodle broth (serves 4)

In this recipe the chicken provides protein to help keep you full for longer and keep your mood steady. The carrot, pepper and spring onions provide fibre and valuable vitamins and minerals. The chilli, ginger and garlic provide disease-preventing phytochemicals.

Ingredients

2 tbsp olive or rapeseed oil
400 g chicken fillets, cut into strips
1 clove garlic, peeled and crushed
5 cm ginger root, peeled and chopped
1 small red chilli, deseeded and finely diced
1 litre chicken or vegetable stock
1 tbsp soy sauce
1 large carrot (about 150 g in weight) cut into matchsticks
1 red pepper, deseeded and cut into matchsticks
8 spring onions, sliced
200 g egg noodles, cooked according to instructions on pack
1 handful fresh coriander leaves

Method

Heat the oil in a large frying pan or wok. Add the chicken strips and fry until they begin to turn golden. Add the garlic, ginger and chilli, and fry for a further minute. Add the stock and soy sauce, and bring to the boil. Add the carrot, red pepper and spring onions. Reduce the heat and simmer until the vegetables are softened (but still retain a slight crunch). Add the noodles and heat through. Serve in bowls, scattered with the fresh coriander leaves.

Liver and onions with leek mash (serves 4)

In this recipe the liver provides protein to keep your blood sugar steady and health-boosting vitamins A, B and C, iron and selenium. The onions and leeks are good sources of vitamin C, folic acid and fibre.

Ingredients
For the liver and onions
600 g calf's liver cut into 2-cm thick slices
4 tbsp plain flour
Freshly ground black pepper
3 tbsp olive oil
175 ml red wine
500 ml hot vegetable stock
2 sprigs fresh thyme
1 bay leaf
350 g carrots, peeled and sliced
2 large onions, peeled and chopped

For the leek mash
500 g potatoes, peeled and cut into chunks
3 tbsp olive oil
2 leeks, thinly sliced
Freshly ground black pepper

Method
Preheat oven to 180°C/350°F/Gas mark 4.

Liver and onions
Place the liver slices onto a plate. Sprinkle with the flour and season

with the freshly ground black pepper. Heat a casserole dish, then add one tablespoon of the olive oil. Add the liver in batches and fry until golden brown. Set aside on a plate. Pour the red wine into the casserole dish used to cook the liver in. Simmer, stirring well to incorporate the particles of liver on the bottom of the dish, until the wine is reduced by a third, then add the stock, thyme, bay leaf and carrots, and season to taste with freshly ground black pepper. Return the liver to the casserole and stir gently, then place in the oven and cook for 30-45 minutes, or until the liver is tender. Heat a frying pan until hot and add the remaining olive oil and onions. Fry the onions for 2-3 minutes, or until golden brown and tender. Set aside and keep warm.

Leek mash

Cook the potatoes in a saucepan of boiling water for 10-15 minutes, or until soft. Drain well then mash with a potato masher until smooth. Heat one tablespoon of olive oil in a frying pan and add the leeks. Fry gently for 3-4 minutes until softened. Season to taste with freshly ground black pepper and add to the mashed potato. Add the remaining olive oil and mix well. Divide the leek mash among four serving plates, placing the liver alongside. Spoon on the fried onions, then pour the red wine gravy over the whole dish.

Mixed bean cassoulet (serves 4)

In this vegetarian recipe the beans provide filling protein and fibre, as well as vitamins and minerals. The butternut squash provides the antioxidant beta-carotene, while the tomatoes provide lycopene. The thyme and bay leaves provide phytochemicals.

Ingredients

1 tbsp olive oil
1 onion, peeled and chopped
2 garlic cloves, peeled and crushed

1 butternut squash, deseeded and cut into 1.5-cm cubes
1 tbsp tomato puree
300 ml vegetable stock
400 g can chopped tomatoes
2 bay leaves
2 sprigs fresh thyme
2 x 400 g cans mixed beans (e.g. kidney, cannellini and pinto beans), drained and rinsed
Freshly ground black pepper

Method

Preheat oven to 200°C/400°F/Gas mark 6. Heat oil in a flameproof casserole dish and gently fry the onion for five minutes until softened. Add the garlic and butternut squash and cook for a further minute, stirring all the time. Stir in the tomato puree then add the stock, chopped tomatoes, bay leaves, thyme and beans. Stir well then slowly bring to the boil. Cover the casserole dish with a lid and cook in the oven for 25 minutes. Serve in bowls with crusty wholemeal bread. Season to taste with freshly ground black pepper.

Gingered rhubarb and honey syllabub (serves 4)

In this recipe the rhubarb provides antioxidants called polyphenols, as well as vitamin K, calcium and both soluble and insoluble fibre. The Greek yoghurt provides protein, calcium and beneficial bacteria.

Ingredients

4 sticks of rhubarb
Juice of an orange
1 tsp ground ginger
3 tbsp honey
4 tbsp low-fat creme fraiche
500 g Greek yoghurt

Method

Wash the rhubarb, then trim off the ends and cut into 1-cm chunks. Put in a saucepan then add the orange juice, ground ginger and 2 tbsp of the honey. Bring to the boil then simmer gently until the rhubarb starts to soften but is still holding its shape. Put four chunks of rhubarb and a little syrup to one side. Spoon the rest of the mixture into the bottom of glass serving bowls and chill. To make the syllabub, blend the low-fat creme fraiche, Greek yoghurt and remaining honey. Spoon the syllabub mixture over the chilled rhubarb, then top each bowl with a chunk of the reserved rhubarb and a drizzle of the syrup.

Date, apple and walnut muffins (makes 15)

In this recipe the wholemeal flour, apple and dates provide fibre and slow-release energy. The walnuts provide healthy fats and protein.

Ingredients

300 g self-raising wholemeal flour
50 g bran flakes, crushed
1 tsp ground cinnamon
15 walnuts, chopped
65 g dates, chopped
1 egg
50 g soft brown sugar
2 tbsp olive or rapeseed oil
250 ml semi-skimmed milk
100 g eating apple, peeled and grated

Method

Preheat the oven to 190°C/375°F/Gas mark 5. In a large bowl, sift together the wholemeal flour, bran flakes and cinnamon. Stir in the chopped walnuts and dates. In another bowl, beat the egg with the soft brown sugar and oil until well mixed, then stir in the milk and grated apple. Pour into the flour mixture and fold in gently, being careful not to over-mix. Spoon mixture into non-stick or muffin-case-lined muffin tins, filling almost to the top. Bake for around 20 minutes, or until a wooden skewer inserted into the middle of a muffin comes out clean and the tops are golden.

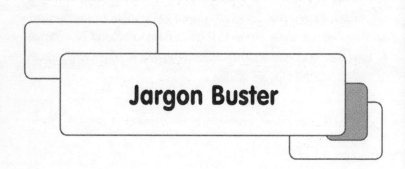

Jargon Buster

Below are explanations of terms used in this book that you may be unfamiliar with.

 Adrenaline – a hormone released by the adrenal glands during the stress response.

Amino acids – organic acids that the body uses in order to make proteins.

Antioxidants – substances thought to neutralise free radicals.

Comfort zone – situations and actions a person feels at ease with.

Cortisol – a hormone released by the adrenal glands during the stress response.

 Dopamine – a neurotransmitter (brain chemical) involved in feelings of pleasure.

 Endorphins – the body's own painkillers.

Free radicals – substances produced by normal chemical reactions in the body and linked to cell damage.

Gamma-aminobutyric acid (GABA) – a neurotransmitter (brain chemical) that promotes calm by reducing brain activity.

Melatonin – the 'body clock' hormone that regulates sleep and waking.

Neurotransmitter – a brain chemical with a role in the transmission of messages from one nerve cell to another. Some neurotransmitters increase brain activity and others reduce it.

Placebo – an inactive substance given to study participants in order to compare its effects with those of a treatment.

Placebo effect – situation where a person taking a placebo feels better because they believe they have received a treatment, and therefore expect to feel better.

Selective serotonin reuptake inhibitor (SSRI) – a type of antidepressant that boosts levels of the 'happy hormone' serotonin in the brain.

Serotonin – a neurotransmitter involved in mood, relaxation, appetite and sleep.

Tryptophan – an amino acid the body uses to make serotonin and melatonin.

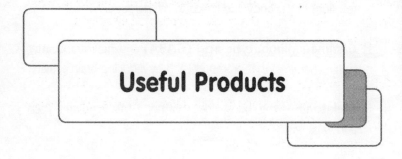

Useful Products

Below is a list of products and suppliers of products that may help to boost confidence. The author doesn't endorse or recommend any particular product and this list is by no means exhaustive.

Bach Calm Official Flower Remedy Shop
Online supplier of Bach Flower Remedies.
Website: www.bachfloweressences.co.uk

Bach Confidence Remedy Balm
An aloe vera gel containing mimulus, water violet, holly and larch, along with neroli and Roman chamomile essential oils; for when you are feeling a little low and lacking self-confidence, or when you need to face a challenge. Apply to pulse points.
Website: www.bachfloweressences.co.uk

Dormeasan
Registered herbal tincture containing valerian and hops, to relieve stress, calm and relax. Provides relief from sleep disturbances caused by stress and worry.
Website: www.avogel.co.uk

ESI Passiflora and Valerian Plus
Alcohol-free liquid extract to aid relaxation and sleep. Contains passiflora (passionflower), valerian, chamomile and other calming herbs.
Website: www.auravita.com

G Baldwin & Co
Herbalist founded in London in 1844. Offers a wide range of herbal supplements, tinctures and teabags.
Website: www.baldwins.co.uk

Healthspan 5-HTP 100 mg
Supplement containing 5-HTP, vitamin C, biotin, niacin, vitamin B6, folic acid and zinc.
Website: www.healthspan.co.uk

Jobar Pedal Pusher Exerciser
Compact pedal pusher exerciser that can be used whilst seated to exercise leg muscles and stimulate circulation in the legs, ankles and feet.
Website: www.stressnomore.co.uk

Kalms
A herbal remedy for the relief of stress, worry and to promote sound sleep. Contains valerian and calming gentian and hops.
Website: www.kalmsstress.com

Napiers Skullcap, Oat and Passionflower Compound
A classic nerve tonic containing a range of calming herbs including skullcap, oats, passionflower and valerian.
Website: www.napiers.net

Nelson's Homeopathic Pharmacy
Homeopathic pharmacy founded in 1860. Sells homeopathic remedies and Bach Flower Remedies online.
Website: www.nelsonspharmacy.com

Prewett's Instant Chicory (100 g)
A caffeine-free alternative to coffee, made from roasted chicory root.
Website: www.prewetts.co.uk

RelaxHerb
Supplement containing pharmaceutical-grade extract of passion flower to relieve stress and worry.
Website: www.schwabepharma.co.uk

Serotone 5-HTP
Supplement containing 5-HTP (50 mg or 100 mg) along with the mineral zinc and B vitamins.
Website: www.highernature.co.uk

Solgar 5-Hydroxytryptophan (5-HTP)
Supplement containing 100 mg of 5-HTP, along with magnesium, valerian root extract and vitamin B6.
Website: www.solgar.co.uk

Stop'n Grow
A bitter-tasting liquid you apply to your nails to stop you biting them.
Website: www.auravita.com

Stressless
Tablets that harness the sedative properties of valerian, hops, skullcap and vervain, to help relieve stress and nervous tension.
Website: www.hollandandbarrett.com

Symingtons Classic Dandelion Coffee (100 g)
Caffeine-free coffee substitute made from dandelion roots.
Website: www.healthstore.uk.com

Tisserand Aromatherapy
This company offers a wide range of good quality essential oils designed to improve health and happiness.
Telephone: 01273 325666
Email: sales@tisserand.com
Website: www.tisserand.com

Vitano
A supplement containing pharmaceutical-grade standardised extract of rhodiola rosea, which can relieve worry, stress and exhaustion.
Website: www.schwabepharma.co.uk

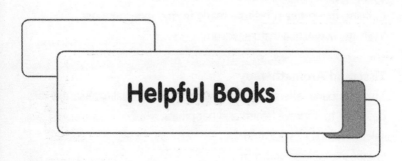

Helpful Books

Harrold, Fiona, *Indestructible Self-Belief: 7 simple steps to getting it and keeping it* (Piatkus, 2011). A compact guide to boosting your self-belief and achieving your full potential.

Jeffers, Susan, *Feel the Fear and Do it Anyway* (Vermillion, 2007). A life-changing guide that shows you how you can become more confident by taking control of your life and stepping out of your comfort zone.

Baumgartner, Jennifer, *You Are What You Wear: What Your Clothes Reveal About You* (Da Capo Lifelong, 2012). This book explains how the clothes you wear are an outward expression of how you feel about yourself and your life, and how giving your wardrobe a makeover can help boost your confidence and aspirations.

Henderson, Veronique & Henshaw, Pat, *Colour Me Beautiful: Change Your Look – Change Your Life: expert guidance to help you feel confident and look great* (Hamlyn, 2010). A useful guide to choosing clothes, make-up and a hairstyle to suit your colouring, shape and style.

Fairley, Josephine & Stacey, Sarah, *Beauty Bible Beauty Steals* (Kyle Cathie, 2009). This book gives you the lowdown on the most effective budget-priced beauty products.

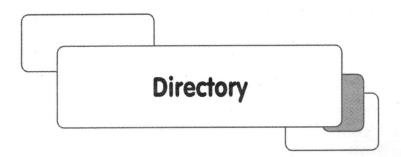

Directory

Below is a list of contacts offering useful information and support for topics and issues covered in this book.

Bigwardrobe.com
Website where you can swap, buy and sell clothes, shoes and accessories.
Website: www.bigwardrobe.com

The British Homeopathic Society
Charitable association that aims to promote homeopathy by providing authoritative information and supporting research and training in homeopathy.
Website: www.britishhomeopathic.org

Citizens Advice Bureau
Helps people resolve their legal, financial, emotional and other problems by providing free, independent and confidential advice. Visit the website for online advice and contact details for your local CAB.
Registered office: Myddelton House, 115–123 Pentonville Road, London N1 9LZ
Website: www.citizensadvice.org.uk

Clothes for Cash
A website that allows you to recycle your clothes, shoes and accessories as well as make some cash and help people in the Third World.
Website: www.clothesforcash.com

Freecycle
An online recycling organisation that aims to reduce waste, save resources and ease the burden on landfill sites, by encouraging people to give and receive unwanted items for free.
Website: www.freecycle.org

Freegle
A recycling organisation that aims to keep anything reusable out of landfill sites by encouraging people to give away and receive unwanted items for free.
Website: www.ilovefreegle.org

Health Supplements Information Service
A service that aims to provide accurate and balanced information on vitamins, minerals and food supplements.
Address: 52a Cromwell Road, London SW7 5BE
Email: info@hsis.org
Website: www.hsis.org

International Stress Management UK
ISMAUK is a registered charity and the leading professional body representing a multi-disciplinary professional health and wellbeing membership in the UK and the ROI. It promotes sound knowledge and best practice in the prevention and reduction of human stress.
Telephone: 0845 680 7083
Email: stress@isma.org.uk
Website: www.isma.org.uk

Medicines and Healthcare products Regulatory Agency
A government agency that is responsible for ensuring that medicines and medical devices work, and are acceptably safe.
Address: 151 Buckingham Palace Road, London SW1W 9SZ
Telephone: 020 3080 6000
Email: info@mhra.gsi.gov.uk
Website: www.mhra.gov.uk

Mental Health Foundation
UK charity which provides helpful information about, and carries out research into, the causes, prevention and treatment of mental health problems, including low self-confidence, low mood and stress. The foundation also campaigns for, and works to improve, services for anyone affected by mental health problems. It takes an integrated approach to mental health that incorporates both social and biological factors. Online resources include downloadable podcasts on stress and relaxation. The charity's Be Mindful campaign offers information on reducing your stress levels by using mindfulness, an online mindfulness course and details of mindfulness courses across the UK.
Address: Mental Health Foundation, London Office, 9th Floor, Sea Containers House, 20 Upper Ground, London SE1 9QB
Telephone: 020 7803 1100
Website: www.mentalhealth.org.uk

Mind
A national charity for people with emotional and mental health problems, including stress, low self-confidence and low mood; offers information and advice online, as well as through a network of local Mind associations that provide counselling, befriending and drop-in sessions, etc.
Address: 15-19 Broadway, London E15 4BQ
Telephone: 020 8519 2122

Mind Information Line: 08457 660163 (local rate, Monday to Friday, 9.15 a.m.–5.15 p.m.)
Email: contact@mind.org.uk
Website: www.mind.org.uk

The Money Advice Service
An organisation that provides advice on a range of financial issues, including managing your money, dealing with debt, savings, mortgages and pensions; the website contains a host of tools and advice to help you take control of your finances.
Telephone: Money Advice Line – 0300 500 5000 (Monday to Friday, 8 a.m.–6 p.m, except bank holidays); typetalk 18001 0300 500 5000
Address: The Money Advice Service, 25 The North Colonnade, London E14 5HS
Email: enquiries@moneyadviceservice.org.uk
Website: www.moneyadviceservice.org.uk

Money Saving Expert
A website dedicated to saving people money on anything and everything, by finding the best deals and beating the system. Created by leading financial journalist Martin Lewis.
Website: www.moneysavingexpert.com

NHS Direct
NHS website that offers an online initial assessment, where you can check your symptoms and get health advice, including advice on mental health issues such as depression and low self-confidence. The website links to NHS Choices, which has a 'healthy living' section with advice on mental wellbeing, including mindfulness. You can also find out about psychological therapy services, such as counselling and CBT, near you. Useful online tools include workplace stress,

mental health and lift-your-mood video walls, where people share their experiences via video clips. There are also blogs and forums on specific health topics (NHS Choices Talk), including mental health issues, such as low self-confidence and low mood.
NHS Stressline: 0300 123 2000 (8 a.m.–10 p.m., seven days a week)
Website: www.nhsdirect.nhs.uk

Really Worried
A website where you can seek or share help and advice on just about any worrying issue.
Website: www.reallyworried.com

Relaxation for Living Institute
A charity which offers information on stress and its effects on the body, as well as relaxation techniques. Also provides a database of Relaxation for Living Institute teachers and relaxation classes across the UK.
Address: Relaxation for Living Institute, 1 Great Chapel Street, London W1F 8FA
Telephone: 020 7439 4277
Website: www.rfli.co.uk

The Society of Teachers of the Alexander Technique (STAT)
Website that provides information about the Alexander Technique, including the latest research, a database of Alexander Technique teachers, and details of courses and workshops across the UK.
Address: 1st Floor, Linton House, 39–51 Highgate Road, London NW5 1RS
Telephone: 0845 230 7828
Website: www.stat.org.uk

The Stress Management Society

The Stress Management Society is a non-profit-making organisation dedicated to helping people tackle stress. The website offers a wealth of information about stress and how to deal with it.

Telephone: 0844 357 8629

Email: info@stress.org.uk

Website: www.stress.org.uk

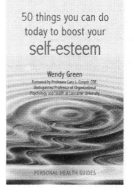

50 THINGS YOU CAN DO TODAY TO IMPROVE YOUR SELF-ESTEEM

Wendy Green

ISBN: 978 1 84953 405 5

Paperback   £6.99

In this easy-to-follow book, Wendy Green explains the lifestyle and psychological factors that can affect your self-esteem, and guides you through the steps you can take to improve your relationship with yourself, offering practical advice and a holistic approach, including simple dietary and lifestyle changes and DIY complementary therapies. Find out 50 things you can do to boost your self-esteem today including:

- Identify the causes of low self-esteem and learn how to manage them
- Choose mood-boosting foods and supplements
- Fit self-esteem enhancing exercise into your daily life
- Use positive self-talk to reduce stress and improve your self-image
- Learn to love the way you look
- Recognise and build on your strengths, talents and achievements
- Find helpful organisations and products

'This book provides practical solutions to enhance people's self-esteem, suggestions that are within everybody's control… listen and engage with its sound advice.'

Professor Cary L. Cooper, CBE, Distinguished Professor of Organizational Psychology and Health at Lancaster University

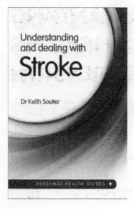

UNDERSTANDING
AND DEALING
WITH STROKE

Dr Keith Souter

ISBN: 978 1 84953 390 4

Paperback   £8.99

It is estimated that there are up to 30 strokes every minute throughout the world.

A stroke can be fatal or disabling, while others are purely temporary with a recovery time of less than 24 hours. Whatever the case, a stroke is always serious and as well as having physical and mental consequences for the sufferer, it can also have a significant effect on other family members.

This book gives the basic information needed to understand what a stroke is, how to spot the risk factors that may contribute to a stroke, and how to take steps to deal with the repercussions, including details on:

- What happens in a stroke
- The different types of stroke
- Stroke recovery and rehabilitation
- Medication and aids and equipment for independent living

Dr Keith Souter is an established medical writer and Fellow of the Royal College of General Practitioners. He is the author of *50 Things You Can Do Today to Manage Back Pain* (ISBN: 978 1 84953 120 7).

UNDERSTANDING AND DEALING WITH DEPRESSION

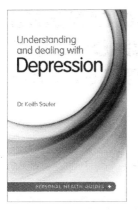

Dr Keith Souter

ISBN: 978 1 84953 391 1

Paperback   £8.99

People suffering from depression can feel helpless and lost, but a basic understanding of the condition can go a long way to helping to treat it and its symptoms.

Depression affects 1 in 5 adults at some point during their lives, and for many people it can seriously affect their quality of life, as well as having a significant effect on family and friends.

This book gives the basic information needed to understand what depression is, how to recognise it, and, most essentially, how to deal with it, including details on:

- Different types of depression
- What depression can feel like
- Medical and holistic ways of treating depression
- Things you can do yourself to control the symptoms

Dr Keith Souter is an established medical writer and Fellow of the Royal College of General Practitioners. He is the author of *50 Things You Can Do Today to Manage Back Pain* (ISBN: 978 1 84953 120 7).

Have you enjoyed this book?
If so, why not write a review on your favourite website?

If you're interested in finding out more about our books, find
us on Facebook at **Summersdale Publishers** and follow us on
Twitter at **@Summersdale**.

Thanks very much for buying this Summersdale book.

www.summersdale.com